Project Elinor

The Illness

10 Steps to Overcoming Any of Life's Obstacles

*How to transform your mind to get through difficult times
and live the happy and healthy life
you deserve to live now!*

Life Recovery Coach NADIA FINLEY

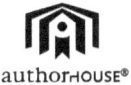

authorHOUSE®

AuthorHouse™
1663 Liberty Drive
Bloomington, IN 47403
www.authorhouse.com
Phone: 1-800-839-8640

First published by AuthorHouse 2/10/2011

ISBN: 978-1-4520-8044-4 (sc)
ISBN: 978-1-4520-8045-1 (hc)
ISBN: 978-1-4520-8043-7 (e)

Library of Congress Control Number: 2010914833

Printed in the United States of America

This book is printed on acid-free paper.

Acknowledgements

I'd like to thank everyone who made this book possible, especially: Anne Marie and Brad Baker from Ekagra Studio B3 Fitness. Andreas Barrett from dre de beroid, Chris Wynia from Chris Wynia Photography, and Carmine Groe from Carmine Groe Photographs. Also my deepest thanks to Nacia Barrett, Mirella Giovenco, Tim LeeLoy, Sabrina Furgiuele, Kerry Colarusso, Mary Tran, Ursula Janicki, Kevin Mercier, Matthew Ribau, and Marc Curcio.

To my family whom I adore: Lara, Erin and Dad.

This book is dedicated to my late mother Elinor, who taught me to live life to the fullest and remain humble along the way. Thank you for teaching me how to be a woman with class, beauty, wisdom and strength. I tip my hat to you for showing your daughters how to stand up for ourselves and to speak up if we want to be heard. Thank you for teaching me that girls can play hockey, be aggressive, practice karate, and yet still wear skirts, put on make-up, and be confident in who we are.

For Aunt Chrissy

"God grant me the serenity to accept the things I
cannot change, courage to change the things I can,
and the wisdom to know the difference."

The Serenity Prayer
Alcoholics Anonymous

CONTENTS

Disclaimer

Any information or advice offered by this book is not intended to provide an alternative to professional medical treatment or to replace the advice of your physician, psychotherapist, or psychiatrist. You should always seek the help of a professional if needed.

The author specifically disclaims all responsibility for any liability incurred as a consequence, directly or indirectly, of the use and application of any of the contents of this book.

PREFACE

This is a book about recovery. It's about recognizing negative circumstances and overcoming them in order to live the happy, healthy life we all deserve to live.

I wrote this book because I know what it feels like to watch my world shatter within a matter of minutes. I know what it's like to feel beside myself, utterly incredulous at how everything can change so quickly, and reeling at the shock of it all. I remember the feeling that I wished I could turn back time because nothing could be worse than the present moment. I will talk more about this later on.

Countless books have been written on the topic of loss. When you walk into a bookstore or library, you can locate hundreds of books focused on helping people overcome anything from failed marriages to crushed self-esteem. Many authors have dedicated countless pages to guiding you through grief, offering ways to make the next chapter of your life easier and perhaps more fulfilling.

Then there are the experts who discuss happiness and what it means to be truly happy. They talk about life transformations and how to begin the quest for contentment. There are wonderful books out there on what happiness means and how to achieve it in all stages of life.

Then, finally, there are the books on nutrition, fitness, and emotional and spiritual well-being. They teach us to live from the inside out, and they stress the importance of eating well and maintaining an exercise routine. They teach us to look inward for the answers to questions that burden us. These books teach us that it is just as important to feed your body with nutrition as it is to feed your mind and soul with good energy.

My book combines all of these different approaches to provide you with holistic strategies for achieving overall wellness. I do not focus on one aspect, but rather the full spectrum of tools for living well. I speak from the heart. I discuss the realities of life's circumstances as they affect all of us in today's hectic world. None of us is exempt from life's struggles, or the pain that comes with them. My theories are based on real-life experience – what I've learned from my own personal suffering and the findings I've collected from people like you, along the way.

In my quest through pain, healing and healthy living, I've learned that we all suffer and that we will continue to suffer. I teach my readers that it's not a matter of trying to avoid sorrow, as sadness is simply a part of life. On the contrary, our suffering builds us and makes us stronger; our pain makes us human and humble. It's when we are at our lowest that we are able to prove how resilient we actually are. We cannot ignore our losses because they will affect us time and time again; we just need to get better at preparing ourselves for them.

The reality is, despite what any of us is going through right now, the desire to be healed is universal. Regardless of the nature of our losses and life struggles, we all suffer and consequently heal in very similar ways.

This book is designed such that you can just pick it up and begin reading the chapter(s) pertaining to you right now. Each chapter is intended to be its own entity; and so you will find that some chapters recap the ideas introduced in others. Be assured these are not redundancies but reiterations of important themes. The 10 steps discussed in this book cover the entire healing process as seen through the lens of Project Elinor. You decide which steps are most relevant to your healing.

This book will help you learn to heal yourself.

INTRODUCTION

*P*roject Elinor is designed to help anyone whose life has been affected by *Illness* but wants to lead a happy, healthy and vigorous life. The definition of an Illness in this program is not necessarily connected to a physical sickness. Illness, as I will explain further in Chapter 1, is a term used to describe our most negative experiences because of what they have the ability to do to each of us — both physically and emotionally. I view the term Illness to mean *any* personal life experience that negatively affects one's well-being.

My most profound Illness occurred when my mother's sudden death set my world reeling. For you, it may also be the loss of a loved one, or perhaps it's a marital or relationship breakdown. Maybe it's financial crisis or job loss. It could also be a matter of lost self-esteem or self-identity.

Regardless of the particular life event through which you have experienced loss, your most profound life experience is affecting your well-being in negative, large-scale ways. Your Illness, or loss, will have become the event against which you compare all other negative life experiences, until you experience something even more profound than this experience.

Throughout this book I will use the term Illness freely. It is important to note that I use the term Illness not necessarily in its traditional sense, but rather to describe your most negative life experience. When I refer to your Illness, I am speaking of what you are suffering from right now. You determine what that is.

I will use myself as an example.

When I was just eight years old, I had begun to wrestle with what would become my first Illness. I was the daughter of an alcoholic mother. I would never invite friends over because I always feared the state in which

I would find her. I was afraid to bring a friend over unannounced in case my mother would wake up from one of her week-long bouts of drinking and sleeping.

I would visit friends at their own homes, or make excuses as to why we could not meet at mine. Forging my mother's signature on class trip authorization forms or report cards became the norm. This was not because my mother was not interested in my education, but because she was often not sober enough to do so.

And so I adjusted. I learned to hide my mother's alcoholism so well that there wasn't a teacher or friend who suspected a thing. As a bright elementary school student, I was socially adjusted on the outside, all the while hiding my Illness on the inside.

When I got older, I learned I was not the only child dealing with alcoholism in the family, and that it was actually quite common. This is not to say that I learned to trivialize my mother's disease, but I did learn that what had been so mentally and emotionally draining on the entire family required acceptance first, and next, a plan for healing.

As I began to accept my Illness, and I entered the world of teenage frenzy, my Illness turned inward, and instead of being consumed with my mother's faults, I became obsessed with my own.

When I was seventeen, my Illness went from hiding my mother's disease to comparing myself and my abilities to those of my two sisters. When I looked to them, I never felt that I measured up. This had a profound impact on my actions and my self-esteem.

I looked at my eldest sister as someone who excelled in anything she put her mind to. She was a gifted art student whose work demonstrated such prodigious talent that family members and friends could admire it for hours. I used to watch her draw and I was amazed at how her hands moved across the page with ease.

Then there was my younger sister. Aside from her quick wit, and her own artistic abilities, she was a perfectionist – and she really *was* perfect – at everything. She made the honor roll every year in high school and received college scholarships.

Then there was me. I was not an artist and I had never seen my name on the honor roll in high school. My goal in school was not to pass every test or achieve high grades; I was more concerned about being on time for baseball practice or making the cheerleading squad.

When it came time to graduate high school, I determined which university I would attend based on the sports I could play there, and which friends were also enrolled. I attended the University of Toronto for five years, unsure of what I would do with my degree once I graduated. When I finished school, both parents were present to see me get my diploma. My mother told me afterwards that while watching the ceremony, my dad had smiled and said, "This is one place I never thought I'd be."

Despite my ability to successfully graduate with an honors degree, I never felt I possessed the talent my sisters had. Both of them had skills that anyone could see; they were able to create things that people could look at and appreciate.

I, on the other hand, did not have any particular talents, or so I felt. There was not one specific thing I could say I was really good at. This feeling was constant. Not only did it have an impact on my self-esteem, it also affected my perception of my own success in the future. I constantly fought with the notion that I was not as smart or talented as my sisters, and that perhaps there was nothing I could do to change this. This Illness remained with me until I was faced with my most profound experience ever: the loss of my mother. Until this time, I was not able to grow and recognize the talents that I was able to offer.

When I was 24, my Illness came to a head. I walked into the house alone and found my mother had passed away while resting on the couch. I later learned that she had died of heart failure. (She had not had a drink for years, having conquered her own Illness quietly but impressively.)

It was a cool evening on March 24th, 2004, and I recall coming home from the gym and entering the house thinking no one was home since all of the lights were off. I walked up the stairs and into the kitchen. Noting how dark the house was, I flipped a few lights on. I walked into the room where my mother was, and while it appeared she was sleeping, there was something strange about this scene. Instinctively, I knew something was wrong because I refused to turn on the lamp right next to her. As I called her name, I leaned over to touch her and felt a certain stiffness in her neck. I couldn't breathe. I ran into the next room and screamed, "Mom! Mom! Mom!" Although I knew something had happened, I had hoped that if I yelled loudly enough, she might wake up. But there was nothing, no response. My mother would not move.

I grabbed a cordless phone, dialed 911, and ran outside in my socks. All I could say to the operator was, "Something is wrong with my mom." I couldn't use the words 'dead' or 'dying'. I was numb.

My father drove up a few moments later, after picking up one of my sisters from work. I ran to the car, but again, could only mutter the words, "Something's wrong" while I pointed in the direction of the house. My dad had hardly parked the car before running up and into the room where my mother was seated on the sofa. I remember running up the stairs after him and watching him give her CPR. I noticed that her fingertips were blue, but I didn't have the heart to tell my father there was no way he was going to save my mother's life.

Moments later, sirens rang as the ambulance, fire truck, and police cruisers stopped in front of our house. I couldn't stay to watch, so instead I paced around outdoors, waiting for a final verdict. My father remained in the house the whole time, while my youngest sister jogged back and forth between us.

Though the whole event felt like several hours, it was really just one or two. I recall one very kind police officer coming over to me to ask if I wanted to see my mother. In a panicky voice I asked, "Why, is she okay?!" He said, "She's gone, but do you want to see her one last time?" I answered 'No' more confidently than I had ever answered anything in my life. Just a few hours earlier, I had seen my mother sleeping on the couch; she was dressed nicely and she had looked so calm and so beautiful. There was no way I was going to alter that image.

To date, nothing has affected me more deeply than that night and the suddenness of my loss. My world has never been the same and I cannot say I've ever even come close to feeling as weak or as shattered as I did on that chilly March evening. No one person has been capable of bringing me to the same low, and no circumstance since has been as profound. Losing my mother is my Illness: it is the greatest loss I have ever known, but it has also shown me the power of my wherewithal.

I have come to think of the term 'Illness' as pertaining to the trauma experienced due to the loss of any precious and beloved person, thing, or idea. Some of us have been affected many times, or perhaps the loss that we consider the most significant changes frequently. Others may not have been affected as often and their most profound loss remains something that happened many years ago. Regardless of whether you are going through something presently, or whether you have experienced something negative many years ago, the particular event remains, by my definition, your Illness.

CHAPTER I

DEFINING YOUR LOSS
AS AN ILLNESS

It is important to use the term Illness for two reasons. The first reason being that your experience is based on your feelings. When you undergo loss of any kind, your body experiences sensations not unlike those caused by an infection or injury. You have a knot in your stomach, and the idea of everyday living can feel overwhelming or exhausting. For months after I lost my mother, normal daily rituals like going to the gym or getting dressed for work seemed exhausting and irritating. It was like I got up every morning feeling under the weather.

Our Illnesses keep us feeling run down, especially when we are in the early stages. The extent of time and emotion that was put into the relationship with whomever or whatever we have lost will impact the duration of our feeling sick or run down, but will also affect its magnitude. For example, if you were to lose your job after two months of service, as opposed to losing a job after eight years, the likelihood is that you will feel more affected by the latter loss because of a greater investment of time and emotion.

Second, understanding the impact of a loss as an Illness allows you to see it as something that is, in a sense, external, objectifiable, and manageable. When you get up on a Monday morning and feel the onset of a cold, you accept it as a viral infection and know that if you take care of yourself and treat your cold, it will be overcome.

Understanding the impact of a loss as an Illness allows you to see it as a thing that is in your power to name (literally, to come to terms with), and therefore, treatable. With time and proper healing, you will get past this stage in your life and begin living the healthy life you know you deserve.

Throughout the course of this book, I will refer to the impact of your loss – whatever that loss may be – as an Illness, or more accurately, *your* Illness. It's also important to note that my definition of loss is wide in scope. Whereas loss is traditionally associated with death, my definition of the word can also mean the loss of a job, relationship, marriage, or friend. Or, perhaps the loss has to do with you personally, in terms of lost self-esteem or self-confidence. Thus, in this book, loss and Illness are closely related. Your loss (which may become your Illness) is anything that you view as a profound negative life experience that you are trying to work through in order to regain health and happiness.

Regardless of whatever negative life event you are experiencing right now, it is important to accept it as an Illness. You may be "sick", but it is within your power to cure yourself.

CHAPTER 2

SEPARATING YOUR ILLNESS FROM YOU

The mind and body are so closely integrated that when something affects one of these, the other must react also. We witness this in everyday life. When you are physically sick, for example, you feel mentally drained, and not up to doing anything that requires much concentration. On the other hand, when you are emotionally hurt (and it's your mind more so than your body that is initially impacted), you will often feel physically drained and unable to take part in anything. Even everyday activities like taking a walk or going to the gym become daunting tasks.

Because our bodies are not equipped to naturally separate our Illnesses from us, we must actively and consciously do this ourselves.

When we first undergo loss our thoughts are consumed with the Illness. Therefore, learning how to separate your Illness from you is especially important in the early stages of loss because we need to know how to live day-to-day while still accepting the mourning process. (We don't only mourn for those who have passed away; we also mourn the loss of a relationship, the loss of a job, and so on). We need to be able to get up in the morning and go to work, or take care of the children, or simply go to the grocery store. This early stage requires that we work with the little strength we have and consciously manage our thoughts. We tell our minds that we will think about our losses (because we know it's impossible to forget them); however, we need to work out a compromise with our mind/body connection where we allow ourselves sporadically to take "mental breaks" from our Illnesses.

An excellent exercise for temporarily separating our Illnesses from us is what I call the "Box Theory". This exercise is not intended to be a means of its own toward forgetting or disregarding an Illness. Instead, it is an exercise we can do to properly organize our thoughts. It allows us to temporarily put away our thoughts and it gives us permission to blot out the "who/what/where/when and why's" of a particular Illness so we can focus on everyday living.

If we don't separate the Illness from ourselves, it will define us, and ultimately it will own every thought we have. We have all experienced this on some level. Think about the last time you were deeply affected by something. You likely thought about it for what seemed like every waking minute of the day.

Even with something small, like an incident at work or a dispute with a friend, we tend to internalize problems and create mountains out of molehills in our minds. To remedy this, we need to envision ourselves outside of the event and away from the circumstance. We need to separate ourselves from our Illnesses.

Take the next moment to try the "Box Theory". Close your eyes and envision a box, any style of box. Now envision the appearance of the box. Is it red, blue, pink, yellow? Is it light, dark, spotted, striped? Now think about its texture. Does it have a grain, like a wooden box, or is it smooth and silky, like a wedding-ring box? Picture your box with a lid that can be opened or closed – maybe it has a handle too.

Next, envision your loss. In my case, this would be the loss of my mother, but perhaps for you it is the loss of a child, a spouse, or perhaps it is a professional loss, like a job, or a relationship loss, like a divorce or break-up.

Maybe it is simply that you have had a bad work week, or a personal dilemma you have found yourself in that consumes your every thought. Regardless of what your Illness is at the present, imagine it in whatever form you desire. Now, with your eyes still closed, picture yourself performing the following: you're physically holding your Illness, opening the box, and placing the Illness inside the box and shutting the lid. Imagine yourself opening and closing the lid several times before allowing yourself to open your eyes. Ensure the box is placed neatly in the back corner of your mind. Envision yourself taking the closed box and placing it in the corner. Now walk back to the forefront of your mind.

Once you have successfully closed the lid on the box with your Illness inside and placed it in the back of your consciousness, take note that this exercise is done as a promise to yourself to temporarily put aside the anxiety or despair caused by your Illness. You are doing this in order to gain back some control over your own mind. It's as though you are saying, "I'm aware you're there, but I don't want to think about you all day today. I want to accomplish things today, and don't want you to interfere. I want 'X' number of hours during which I won't think about you. You will stay in this box until then." Any time you begin to notice the thought coming back into your mind, actively concentrate on the box (its color, shape, and texture) as a reminder of the commitment you've made with yourself. The promise shall be kept until 'X' hours have passed (you determine the timeframe that is suitable for you). Until then, the box remains closed.

This exercise is particularly important in the initial stages of loss because it is meant to bandage the Illness versus trying to heal you completely. At the early stages of your Illness, you need to take small yet significant steps towards your healing. This exercise operates on the principle that, at the early stages of healing, it is impossible to completely forget or disregard an Illness, thus it helps you find temporary relief so you can function more normally right away.

Recognizing your loss as an Illness and separating it from you allows you to see it as something that does and can exist with or without you. It's an extension of you; it does not define who you are. Too many of us get caught up in all the extremities of the world, whether good or bad, and allow ourselves to believe that these outside factors are a part of us.

For example, you may be a parent, an employee, a sister or brother, a husband or wife, or a friend to certain people. When you are asked to describe yourself, you're quick to acknowledge your relationships or your position at the workplace. Rarely do you state who *you* are, but instead who you are in relation to other people or other things.

By defining yourself as an extension of outside factors, you're not recognizing your existence on its own first. You are seeing yourself and your reason for being as a result of various external relationships. Of course, it's important for you to be proud of these different relationships – indeed they contribute to who you are – but it's also critical to recognize yourself independent of them. If you continue to define yourself as an extension of outside factors, you will inevitably remain vulnerable to everything that happens to you. Rather than seeing yourself living through different experiences, you will identify yourself as a victim to situations. In essence, you will envision the circumstance or experience first, and yourself second.

You must always see yourself (by which I mean your very core) as the only thing that defines you. You are yourself first. Everything else, whether it be your relationships or circumstances, are simply people and events in your life that add color to your world. You allow them to attribute happiness or sadness to your life. They do not define your happiness or sadness.

Allow me to use myself as an example. I am Nadia Finley *first*, who is also sister to two artists, daughter to my parents, and life coach to my clients. I may have lost my mother, just as you may have lost your job, your spouse, or a good friend. However, you are still *you*, just as I am still me. As long as I am a breathing entity, I will always be me, and regardless of what happens, that cannot change. If I lose my status with respect to any of these relationships, I am still myself first and that will never change.

Recognizing yourself outside of, and separate from, your relationships allows you to be defined by your own values and your own vision first. (The ability to recognize this will help you when practicing the "Box Theory", because you understand the notion of separating yourself from everything and everyone around you). Therefore, you are better equipped to accept potential change in any of those relationships and you are less likely to feel victimized by things beyond your control.

The notion of separating everything from you (this includes your physical extremities like your body) will take time. However, it's a liberating, powerful feeling once you have accomplished the ability. Suddenly, anything from how you view your body and weight to the death of a loved one becomes something that you observe from the outside with reason and compassion, versus from the inside with a wide range of uncontrolled emotion.

Consider the following statements to exemplify the difference between YOU and your extensions:

I <u>have</u> friends. My friends are not me.
I <u>have</u> a job. My job is not me.
I <u>have</u> a partner. My partner is not me.
I <u>have</u> experiences. My experiences are not me.

All of the above relations reaffirm the notion that the people, circumstances, and experiences in our lives do not define who we are. We experience life with them, or through them, not *because* of them. If any of these outer experiences turn negative, and become your Illness, being able to separate yourself from them is essential to your recovery.

Ask yourself what your extensions are. List them. Do you view them as outside of you, or do they define who you are? One of the best ways to distinguish if you allow outside factors to define or control you, is to list all the things that are important to you and rank them. Then ask yourself: "If I were to lose the first item on this list, how would I feel?" And more importantly, "Why would I feel this way?"

Consider the list below:

- Children
- Appearance
- Career
- Partner

- Education
- Friends
- Social life
- Health

How would you arrange these items? Be honest. There is no right or wrong order to this list. If you state your career before your children or your partner, you are not saying that you don't love your family, but rather, that your career at this point in your life, is where most of your energy is invested. Review the list and your rankings. The items on the top of the list are those that best describe you.

Assume you have all eight items on your list and an old acquaintance who has not seen you in a while asks, "How's everything? What's going on in your life?" What is your initial response? Assuming you will touch on a number of the items, what strikes you as most important? Is it your career status? Do you tell them about your new Vice President position before anything else? Or is it your relationship(s)? You may have gotten married since you last saw the person asking. Perhaps it is your appearance. Maybe you lost twenty pounds and are proud to tell the story! Or maybe it's your children, one of whom began kindergarten.

Regardless of how your list unfolds, the point is what's on top of the list. And despite what it is, if you were to lose it or if it were to significantly change, what would that do to your overall well-being? If the answer is inconceivable and you can't ever imagine your life without this "outside factor," then you need to re-arrange your thoughts. You need to recognize that everything and everybody is outside of you and that you are *you* with or without them. This is not to suggest that you should be able to live just fine without those dearest to you; however, recognizing people, careers, and social status as extensions of you reiterates the power, resilience, and confidence that lies within each of us if we choose to see it. When you see yourself as separate from your extensions, you learn to love them for what they are versus how they define you. You are then less likely to want to control these outside factors or feel victim to them if they change or move away.

Next, consider your *Lower Self* and *Higher Self* when separating your Illness from you. Be aware of which state of mind you spend most of your time in. When you practice the "Box Theory," be conscious of what you are identifying yourself with. Is it your *Ego* (Lower Self), or your *Intuition* (Higher Self)? We each have both, but unfortunately most of us live our day-to-day lives identifying ourselves with our Lower Self.

Identifying with our Lower Self keeps us in the state of mind where we define our success and happiness by outside factors such as our careers, our bank accounts, the lives of others, and our physical appearance. This kind of mentality will undoubtedly make separating our Illnesses from us difficult to do because we've made "outside factors" the basis for our happiness. Consider my Illness, for example. If I were to remain in victim mode, feeling cheated by this awful experience, how would I ever be able to separate my mother's death from me? That kind of mentality would leave me comparing my life to those of others who were fortunate enough to grow old with both parents. I would be wrongfully making her death 'a part of me', a part of my expectations in life. Instead, I needed to view her unexpected death as an extremely difficult experience that was <u>outside of me</u> and that with time I would overcome.

The Ego drives us to compare our lives to those of others, leaving us feeling inadequate or incomplete. Though we have the choice to live life via our Higher or Lower Self, much too often swayed by our greedy, stress-inducing society, we tend to opt for the latter.

Unfortunately it's not until we experience our Illnesses, that we tend to see the importance of identifying ourselves through our Higher Self. We may lose a loved one or go through a sudden breakup, when suddenly we see how life can change so suddenly and how important our health and happiness truly are. Identifying with your Higher Self is when we see life through our core values, and when we see people (including ourselves) as loving, complex beings regardless of any outside attributes. Living through your Higher Self will always bring you happiness. Living through your Lower Self may give you temporary pleasure, but any happiness it brings cannot be sustained because the Ego lives in a fragile state of fear.

So what does this mean in the realm of loss?

If you are identifying yourself with the wrong state of mind, you will undoubtedly see any Illness as happening to you, rather than around you. Identifying with your Ego will have you thinking about what other people might think of you, or how you failed yourself or those around you. Identifying with your Ego will inevitably connect you to the list we discussed earlier (the list of outside factors, circumstances or people that you should not identify yourself with because they are separate from you).

Identifying with your Intuition or Higher Self, on the other hand, allows you to accept yourself and your intrinsic values that are driven by love and self-respect. Your Intuition promotes self-love and makes you feel connected to something larger than yourself (I am not necessarily referring to religion, but rather acknowledging that you are not the center of the universe). Higher Self identification allows you to be separate from outside circumstances because you are driven by your core rather than your Ego.

Choosing to live in accordance with your Higher Self enables you to live with a state of mind that is peaceful and not controlling. Your Higher Self focuses on the notion that we live in a complex world with an array of complicated, sometimes contradictory people and events. It understands that life isn't fair, and that we shouldn't seek revenge for that reality. Your Higher Self simply allows you to see that experiences (both good and bad) happen *around you* – and that they do not *define you*.

Separating our Illnesses from ourselves is what we need to do in order to move past a particular loss. Similar to a disease invading the human body, our Illnesses attack our self-esteem and overall welfare. Should a disease become a part of us, it can spread quickly. Contrarily, when we envision our Illnesses as separate from ourselves, we can become protected from the very sicknesses that can destroy our physical and emotional well-being.

CHAPTER 3

UNDERSTANDING THE FEELINGS ASSOCIATED WITH YOUR ILLNESS

Next it's important to understand the feelings associated with your Illness, and appreciate that we cannot properly get past our particular Illnesses without first finding peace within ourselves for our loss.

As emotional beings, we experience feelings that create the illusion of a trap, leaving us feeling like we can't move forward. Rather than trudging ahead, we experience a 'pulling' sensation in every direction: up, down, and sideways. The slightest thing can alter our moods and turn a seemingly pleasant day into a flurry of uncontrollable thoughts and emotions.

In many cases we feel like a slave to our emotions, with someone else dictating how we feel. When I lost my mother I recall feeling very short-fused. Shortly after her death, I was in a parking lot when a teenage boy yelled some juvenile remark at me in front of his friends. I was minding my own business, so his comments were completely uncalled for – and were done simply to get a reaction from his friends. Had this not happened so closely after my mother's passing, I would have likely dismissed the comment altogether, chalking it up to the oversized egos of teenage boys.

At this particular time in my life, however, a comment like this put me right over the edge. I got out of my car, walked straight up to the boys, and I began to yell. I'm not quite sure what came out of my mouth – because I'd lost control– but I scolded them for their obnoxiousness. The boys appeared shocked and embarrassed as I walked back to my car and drove away.

When I got back into the car I felt an overwhelming sense of discomfort. I was twenty-four years old and I had just needlessly made a scene in a parking lot in front of a group of boys ten years younger than me. In the course of 20 minutes I had gone from taking a leisurely drive to the store, to feeling complete rage, and finally, experiencing embarrassment and guilt. I felt crazy. I began to think I had some sort of chemical imbalance in the brain: Why was it that I could be set off into rage or tears at any moment?

As I've since learned, that 'crazed' feeling I experienced is actually quite common when we begin to cope with a new Illness. The lack of control we feel over our emotions at this time is normal. This is not to say that my actions were acceptable, or that any of our actions are ever excusable as a result of our losses, but it's important to understand that when coping with extreme circumstances, we are not our usual, grounded selves and we forget the control we have over our emotions.

Five of the most common feelings that I have associated with an Illness are anger, guilt, sadness, fear, and denial. Though the list of emotions experienced may be fuller, I have outlined these five different states of emotion as the most significant. Each of these feelings is tied closely to your development in your journey through loss and it's important to know when or why you're feeling a particular way.

- **Anger** is the number one factor for slowing down the healing process. Through working with most of my clients, I've found this to be the case because anger gives us a false sense of empowerment in a situation where we feel very out of control. ("My mother died and now won't see her grandchildren!"; "I am angry that my employer let me go after 10 years of service!"; or "I am furious that my wife left me for another man!")

- **Guilt** gives us an excuse to simmer. It's a kind of self-punishment we perform when we do not take action or make decisions. ("Though my happiness is at stake, I'm going to stay in this unhealthy marriage for the sake of my children"; or "I'm going to remain at this job even though I hate it, because I would disappoint my family otherwise.")

- **Sadness** occurs when we mourn not only the specific set of events but also for the life we could have had. We mourn everything surrounding the person or circumstance that we've lost, whether it's positive or negative. ("I am saddened that my unfaithful spouse has abandoned me"; or "I am upset that I lost the job I wasn't happy with.")

- **Fear** is a learned behavior based entirely on past events or presumptions about the future. Being afraid is completely based on choice. We feel afraid when we do not live in the moment, but rather, focus on the past or future. ("I fear a life without my husband because I *presume* life alone is unstable, even though I've never experienced it.")

- **Denial** occurs when we are so hurt or disillusioned by an event that we believe it hasn't actually happened. Sometimes we refuse to envision the future in a different light with the changes that we didn't plan for, and therefore, we delay the healing process by living in a "made-up" or unreal world.

Becoming aware of the reasons as to why you are feeling a particular way and actively trying to change this negative state of mind is crucial to your healing process. You may feel some or all of the above emotions, and not in any particular order. Recognizing your feelings and allowing yourself to feel them, as opposed to suppressing them, is a wonderfully empowering feeling. It's okay to cry and feel sad. The key is not to ruminate and get stuck in these feelings.

How do our feelings work in relation to our minds? And more importantly, how do they work in connection to our Illnesses?

Think about it: Life can be understood in three time-related states. First there is the past, encompassing everything that has already happened and <u>cannot be changed</u>. Second, there is the future, and although it is unknown, you can help to shape it, depending on your viewpoint. And finally, there is the present, the moment you find yourself in right now – the moment in which you have complete control over your actions and reactions.

Therefore, if you break up these three life phases, and separate them equally, it becomes clear that approximately 66% of our contentment and well-being lies in our direct control and the attitudes of emotions we choose to have. Only one-third of our life (namely our past) cannot be changed. Everything else can be influenced by you!

What this means is that although we may feel out of control while coping with an Illness, we possess the power to choose how to react to outside influences. Our choices are simply our interpretations of certain situations.

I will use myself as an example. On the night I lost my mother, and for some time afterward, I felt an overwhelming kind of pain. This emotion was often coupled with feelings of anger, resentment, or fear. Though I wasn't aware of it at the time, I chose to experience these feelings based on an event that I deemed devastating.

However, years later, having recovered from my Illness, I can gladly say that the emotions I felt while coping with my mother's loss are no longer as painful. This is not to say that I am not saddened when I think of my mother's death, but rather that I don't experience the same sense of pain that I did when I first lost her.

I chose my feelings based on my interpretation. My mother's death is just as true today as it was when I first lost her, and she is just as much physically gone today as she was then. However, though the event remains the same, my interpretation of it has changed and therefore my feelings have also. Today I'm utilizing the 66% of my total happiness and well-being, and I am choosing to grow from the loss of my mother and not interpret the situation as devastating or unjust. I'm focusing on each present moment and maintaining a positive outlook for the future.

Understanding the choice we have in interpreting situations and consequently our emotions related to them, is just as important as understanding that regardless of those choices, emotions are not constant. Even if you were to decide not to do anything with the emotion you are feeling right now, that feeling won't remain forever – not for anyone. Generally speaking, we are never in any mood – good or bad – constantly.

You're probably wondering: Why would you work on choosing your reactions, if emotions cannot remain forever anyway? If it's human nature not to feel sad, angry, guilty or fearful all of the time, why actively try to change it? Won't it happen anyway?

The simple answer to this question is: "yes". Because emotions aren't constant, they technically will subside into another emotion with or without your willingness to actively change them. But is that good enough?

Though you can surrender to your emotions, why would anyone choose to do so? If you have the ability to consciously change a negative state of mind into a more positive one while coping with your Illness, why wouldn't you want to? Why would you simmer in a negative state of mind?

When I lost my mother, my feelings fluctuated constantly. As exemplified in the story of the teenage boys in the parking lot, I felt like my emotions were running rampant and I had no control. I was a prisoner of my state of mind. How I felt at any given moment would determine how I acted.

Understanding that this kind of emotional fluctuation may be inevitable, we are left with a choice. We can let them be, and wait for them to subside, or we can recognize them for what they are – namely a perspective on a particular event or circumstance – and we can choose to change them if they hinder our well-being. You may not choose your loss, but you can choose your perspective on that loss and ultimately the magnitude of the feelings associated with it.

Therefore, it's not your partner leaving you, your employer firing you, or your mother's death that is making you angry, sad, or upset; it's your perception of the circumstance that's making you feel this way. And until you recognize the power you have to choose how you're going to interpret such events, you will always assume that life is happening *to* you.

So how do you change your emotions? How do you *choose* a more positive state of mind?

First, you need to give yourself time to recognize what emotion you are feeling and whether it's worthy of any attention. Often when coping with our Illnesses, we'll feel a quick rush of emotions. Whether they're good or bad, they can be temporary and thus not worthy of much thought.

It's the feelings that seem to linger, or those that are frequent, that we need to take notice of. When you're simmering in a negative state of mind, you haven't yet made the connection between choice and emotional well-being and you need to start. You need to pick apart your Illness to understand exactly *why* you are feeling the way you are and *why* you feel you have no choice in the matter. You need to know what you are ruminating over.

List the following questions in your journal:

- What is your Illness?
- What about your Illness makes you angry?
- What about your Illness makes you sad?
- What about your Illness makes you afraid?

Be as descriptive as possible with your answers. If you have more questions to add to the above list, be sure to do so, and answer them accordingly. Assume no one is reading this or ever will. What do you notice about your written responses? Are your feelings tied to your Illness directly, or do they pertain to everything *around* the event or circumstance?

Consider my client Joe's answers:

What is your loss?

My wife Ellen left me.

What about your loss makes you angry?

She promised to be with me forever.
We shared a home together.
She's with another man already!

What is it about your Illness that makes you sad?

I am alone.
I failed at making this relationship work.
My dream of a successful marriage is ruined.

What about your Illness makes you afraid?

I don't know how I'll survive on my own financially.
I am worried about what people will say.
I am afraid that I will be alone forever.

Once you have listed all of your answers to these questions, take a step back and evaluate them. Do you see a trend? If your answers mirror any of those above, your feelings are not connected to your Illness, but rather are extensions of your Illness. Where you believe you are mourning a particular loss, in most cases you are actually mourning everything around the loss, and not the loss itself.

In the above example, where Joe was left by his wife Ellen, Joe is not mourning his wife, but rather everything she represents. He's mourning the loss of an ideal happy marriage. He's equating happiness to being with Ellen and equating sadness to being single. He's afraid that being single now means he will be alone forever.

Once we distinguish the reasons why we are feeling a particular way, it becomes much more evident that our feelings are often tied to extensions of our losses and not the Illness itself. Where we might *assume* our Illness is making us feel a certain way, it may actually be our own interpretations of how life needs to be that is making us sad, frightened, or angry. As if happiness is achieved through one equation only.

Understanding where your feelings are coming from, and accepting that they're magnified because of your own presumptions can grant back to you some of the emotional control you may have lost. I'm not suggesting that you will not mourn your Illness, and feel different emotions as a direct result of your Illness because you will. However, I am simply clarifying that as emotional beings, we worsen our state of mind by over-thinking and assuming there is a direct correlation between what we have lost and what we wish we had. Though the two *may* be related they are not identical!

In the above example, where Joe and Ellen have broken up, one can confidently conclude that the relationship was not healthy. Though Joe may not have wished to end the marriage, Ellen acknowledged that she was no longer happy for different reasons and wanted to leave the relationship. Assuming that they had both put some sort of effort into the relationship, and tried fixing it at one point or another, the relationship seemed to have lost a healthy foundation. Whether there was constant fighting, or a lack of communication, the relationship wasn't fulfilling for either person. Although Joe is certainly saddened by the loss of his wife, he is also simply grieving the loss of a romantic view of his marriage. In truth, the foundation of this marriage had been weakening for some time, until finally one party left the marriage altogether. Ultimately, Joe does not really want to be with Ellen; he wants to be with the Ellen <u>who wants to be with him</u>. And as long as the latter is not the case, it's not Ellen he's mourning, but everything she represents.

Though interpreting and deciphering feelings can be difficult, particularly at the initial stages of loss, it's important to find the time to do so. Once you realize that your different emotions are a direct result of extensions of your loss, and not your Illness itself, it becomes easier to interpret your situation differently and feel happier.

Remind yourself of the following:

- You own your definition of happiness
- There is not one single definition of happiness
- Happiness is a feeling that is not given to you by a person or job, it is something you give yourself
- You determine your own emotional well-being; your emotional well-being does not determine you
- Your emotions are a direct result of your perceptions and interpretations
- Once you positively change your perceptions, your emotions will positively change as well

- People and circumstances in our lives can contribute to our happiness, but they do not define it
- When loss occurs, recognize the emotions that are a *direct* result of your loss, and those that are connected to extensions of your loss. (How often are you confusing the two?)

Recognizing what you are feeling and the reasons you are feeling a certain way helps the healing process. Not only can it give you clarity, it can also help you discern the feelings that are not related to your loss at all. Once you define happiness, for example – happiness outside of a particular relationship or career – you'll inevitably own your state of well-being. And rather than being a victim to your emotions, you'll be a creator of them.

CHAPTER 4

CONCENTRATING ON THE MOMENT AND LEARNING HOW TO LIVE IN THE PRESENT

Have you ever tried to identify your life's best moment? Have you truly thought about it – have you narrowed it down to a particular day or a specific event? Perhaps it was the day you got married or the day you had your first child. Maybe it was the day of your high-school or college graduation, or when you landed that important job. Whatever it was, ask yourself this: Were you aware that you were experiencing your best moment ever? Were you aware that you were having the time of your life?

If your answer is "no" – and for many people it is "no" – you're not living in the present. Instead, your best moments are simply memories, and they're long behind you. It's a sad reality, but most people get married, have children, and experience many great things, but they rarely stop to appreciate everything they have as it is happening. Unfortunately, however, we are very quick to define the lowest points of our lives, and we are able to recall these moments quite vividly.

In the realm of loss, the ability to live in the current moment is crucial for our development. You have just been confronted with an unexpected circumstance, and your thoughts are all over the place. You're panicking. You're overwhelmed. You're frustrated. Depending on the event that has just taken place, you are likely caught up in worry about your own life or the lives of those around you. Maybe you are even concerned about futile things – like what other people are thinking. Your mind is frenzied and you need to find the stop button quickly. But how do you do this?

First, you must find acceptance. You need to tell yourself that you are okay, even if you do not believe it. Regardless of the situation you have found yourself in, you do possess the ability to deal with it right now as best you can if you choose to. Our ability to accept any situation, or even to thrive in it, is entirely possible and is completely within our control. It's a variety of external influences that misinform us, suggesting that unless we are 100% happy all of the time, we are not truly happy. This leads us to believe that happiness and enjoyment *can* be had 100% of the time, and if you are experiencing anything less, then you must be an unhappy person.

The fact is, life is full of ups and downs, and learning to accept this and embrace all of these different moments will allow you to also accept any obstacle along the way. When you live in the moment and stop predicting the future or rehashing the past, you begin to appreciate the current moment, even if it's not your moment of choice. It's like reading a book. Chapters can take us through various peaks and valleys in a single story. Perhaps one chapter is bursting with happiness and joy, and the next is full of sadness and grief. Regardless, you don't stop reading the book; instead you read through the chapters, taking one page at a time, embracing the different moods because it's the highs and lows that make up the story.

When we are affected by Illnesses, we must see them through, just as we do the chapters of a book, with its highs and lows. We need to embrace each moment, just as we do each page, and learn to live in the present, despite whether this feels really good or not. We don't skip the sad or frightening chapters in a book, so why would it be any different in our own lives? Why would you feel the need to skip over and ignore these chapters of your life if you wouldn't consider doing so while reading a book? These bumps in the road – our Illnesses, though difficult, to say the least – ultimately help us define ourselves. They're actually necessary stepping-stones for the next chapter in your life. It's not until we encounter each particular moment, or new life event, that we are more appreciative of the people (and things) that we do have in our lives.

A great way to live in the present is through daily journal-writing. It is a fantastic way to freely write and go beyond your most obvious thoughts without being judged or censored. With each entry you must allow yourself to brainstorm freely and without reservation. Assume no one will ever read it and that spelling and grammar are completely irrelevant.

Start your entry with this sentence: "When I got out of bed this morning, I felt _____". Expand on this feeling and describe your day as it unfolded. Be as detailed as possible and try to write without pausing, so there is a constant flow of feeling and productivity. When you stop to think, you risk ruminating and thus distorting your true feelings about that particular moment.

Your initial entries will likely sound like a string of run-on sentences with no particular direction or substance. As you continue to write in your journal daily, the entries may not flow together like chapters from a book; however, they will illustrate the overall tone of the life you're living.

When I first started my journal entries after my mother passed, my entries were highly emotional. I filled pages with questions as to why my mother was taken from me and where she was. I spoke about my father and how I desperately wanted him to overcome this hardship, and that I would do anything to make that happen. Some entries were written while I was in tears, and others were written in bouts of frustration and anger.

As time progressed, and the power of my Illness lessened, my journal entries were far less distressing in tone; instead they became much more inquisitive in nature. Whether I was writing about the direction of my life, my relationships, or my career, my entries were for the most part upbeat and cheerful.

Journal writing can help you live in the present and appreciate today because it prompts you to see the big picture. After having written in your journal for a few weeks, you can begin to assess the progress of your healing by asking yourself the following questions: What is the tone of my journal? Am I constantly wasting my days complaining about others, or do I dwell on situations outside of my control? Am I worrying about the future more than being excited to see what it brings? If a stranger were to pick up my journal, would they learn about someone with a balanced life full of ups and downs, or a string of negative thoughts and complaints?

The attention that you give to your journal-writing will not only rid yourself of pent-up emotions brought on by your Illness, but it will also allow you to track progress and see whether an excess of negativity is ruling your daily life. Journal-writing allows you to appreciate the moment you find yourself in right now. Be keenly aware of whether your entries are focused on the past or future, and ask yourself if this 'rehashing' or 'predicting' is serving you well.

Trust is another key factor in living in the present. Step back and trust that you will heal and things will fall into place as they should. We live in a society that teaches us to secure our future as early as possible, as if we are somehow in control of our own fate. Whether it's the idea of getting married, having children, or putting money into your retirement fund, we learn very early on that certain things should happen because without them we will be unhappy or dissatisfied.

Such assumptions however, beg the questions: If my "plans" for the future don't unfold as anticipated, am I destined to live a life of unhappiness and despair? What if they do happen, but change course unexpectedly? Who plans for divorce on a wedding day, or expects to be fired the first day they walk into a new job? What about the heart-wrenching stories of parents forced to deal with a terminally ill child? Such circumstances can cripple us, making us feel as though our world is coming to an end, and yet in no way could they have been predicted and thus, detoured.

If such situations do arise – and no one is exempt from the possibility of this – you may ask how one learns to *trust* that everything will eventually be as it should. How do we embrace painful events and learn to trust the moment as a circumstance that can be managed? How do we learn to trust that this experience will actually help us to grow?

The answer: Consider the possibilities.

When one door closes, how can you find another way out? When your marriage or relationship has failed, what door will lead you to love again? When you lose your job after years of service, what door will allow you to seek security and prestige in the workplace again? When you're coping with the death or illness of a loved one, what door will help you find the strength and courage to survive?

Trusting the moment means acknowledging that your world – as painful as it may feel to be in that world – never has only one door. When you step back and see the full picture, you can put aside the notion of "what should have been" and begin to see the different doorways to happiness - the doorways that are in front of you right now.

Let us consider the analogy of a fork in the road. For the longest time you may have thought your life was going along a very straight and smooth road. If someone asked about your future, you were likely more concerned about its lack of excitement than any sudden change it could have in store, let alone any tragic experience it might contain ahead. Yet when faced with an Illness you feel as though you've reached a dead-end. The path you were comfortably traveling seems to have been cut short and you feel as though you have nowhere to turn. You cannot see past your Illness, because it was never planned. Or worse, it was never supposed to happen to you. Somehow, you were supposed to be exempt.

Unfortunately no one is immune to what I deem Illnesses, and living in the moment allows you to embrace different situations as is, good or bad. It means recognizing that there is always more than one door and that things may or may not happen as planned. When presented with a sudden fork in the road, you will want to ask yourself the following questions to help guide you down your new path – the path of the current moment.

What is your new door?

- Do I have more time to do things I have always wanted to do?
  My relationship has ended and I want to use my free time to explore new and exciting things.

- What skills can I refine for a new career?
  I lost my job and so I want to take this opportunity to enter a field I have always wanted to pursue.

- What sport can I try? Which gym should I join?
  I want to lift my self-esteem and self-confidence by setting goals to get fit and meet new people.

- What family members or friends would I like to reconnect with?
  I suddenly lost a close family member or friend and I now realize how short life can be. I want to reach out to those I care about.

- What places have I always wanted to see?
  A family member is ill and I want to experience as much of the world as I can with them while we are both on this earth together.

Answering the questions above will help you to look beyond yourself, and consider the world of opportunities that your Illness can create. (We will go into greater depth as to what our Illnesses can teach us in Chapter 8.)

If you find yourself unable to consider the positive possibilities of your Illness at this time, take comfort in knowing that you will deal with the circumstance at hand. If you find that you do not yet possess the strength to look past your Illness, give yourself permission to take the time to heal.

Sometimes we simply need to remind ourselves that though it will be painful, we will undoubtedly heal as more time passes. It's the feeling of giving in to a higher power and saying, "I don't know what to do; however, I believe I can deal with this." In saying this to yourself, you can focus on your healing versus your Illness.

Cutting out the chatter or the noise in your mind is imperative to living in the moment. The constant 'talk' that fills our minds throughout the day is commonly devoted to regrets about the past or worries about the future. The moment you are in right now simply doesn't have fear or regret attached to it because such feelings are tied to the notion of time. Therefore, if you think 'in the moment' and not in the past or future, you will live in a 'timeless' state that does not drag negative emotions into it.

So why do you feel happy or sad in a given moment?

You feel different emotions in a particular moment based on the series of thoughts you connect to a certain situation. You are happy when you are with your husband or wife because of the pleasant thoughts you have that relate to past events shared together. You are frightened in a fast-moving car because of the thoughts you have of what could happen if you were to get into an accident. You are sad when someone dies because of the past memories you shared together.

All of these feelings, whether pleasant, fearful or sad, are associated with the past or future. You are the catalyst for bringing them into the current moment.

Being aware is the key to cutting out the chatter and noise that fills your mind on a continuous basis. I'm not suggesting you stop thinking (though it is possible to be above thought through practice and meditation); I am simply asking you to be aware of your thoughts. Take note of the moment you are in by being aware of how connected you have made yourself to certain thoughts (and consequently, emotions). Learn to disconnect even if, initially, it's only for a few moments at a time.

Are you aware of the present moment? Do you see how many of your thoughts are associated with the past or future and therefore, do not serve you in the present moment? Do you see how you are the one who brings memories of the past, or presumptions of the future, into your current state – where they do not belong if they do not serve you well?

Living in the present moment is closely connected to your perceptions of the world because it teaches us how to disconnect the past from the future. Though different circumstances may be out of your control, how you perceive them will always be managed by you. Once you recognize that the perceptions you choose affect your mood, and in turn your actions, you will likely be very careful with your choices in the future.

Consider the two situations below, both of them which stemmed from the loss of a loved one:

Scenario 1: Death of a husband

Perception: "I will never get into another relationship again."
Mood: Sad/ depressed
Action: Stay at home with no desire to get back into a social scene
Outcome: Remain single and disconnected to the outside world

Scenario 2: Death of a husband

Perception: "With time, I know I will heal and grow from this."
Mood: Hurt/ hopeful
Action: Spending time with friends (and perhaps open to dating with time)

Outcome: Potential for new relationships (maybe even romantic relationships)

In recognizing the rationale, it becomes obvious that mastering our minds is completely within our control. Though the circumstance, namely the death of a partner in the example above, may be out of our control, the moods, perceptions, actions, and consequently the outcomes are, indeed, within our power. You choose your state of living through your own interpretation of the world around you. As long as you remain in victim-mode, where you believe things happen to you, and that you cannot help but feel the way you do as a result of outside factors, you will always feel unsafe and completely controlled by your situations and circumstances. When you allow noise and chatter to invade your mind, you will remain a victim to your fears. When you truly understand this, and appreciate that negative circumstances do not have to define us, the secret to living happily can never be taken from you.

CHAPTER 5

ASKING YOURSELF WHAT YOU WANT OUT OF THIS CIRCUMSTANCE AND MASTERING THAT GOAL

B ecause you are going through a particularly painful experience, there is no better time than the present to master something within your control.

This step in the recovery process is all about *you*. Now is when you get to be "selfish" and determine a personal goal that you are going to see materialize. Your focus is on moving past the Illness. It's time to focus on a better you.

Your life is different now, so it's important to take this opportunity to become good at something, or simply *better* at something that interests you.

First, ask yourself the following: What are your goals, and what has kept you from accomplishing them?

Do you want to drop ten or twenty pounds? Would you like to go back to school? How do you feel about traveling through Europe? Are you thinking of joining a sports or social club? These might be the kinds of goals you would like to reach. Or maybe it's simpler than any of these: perhaps you would like to try to set aside 20 minutes each day for personal reflection.

Whatever your goal is — you choose it, you own it, and you achieve it. There is no better time than right now to focus on your self-betterment, so let go of all your negative "I can't do this" talk, and take action. You've just been fueled with a ton of emotion, albeit negative energy, so let's take that, and invest it toward a goal that is completely about you!

Some of the best times of my life have revolved around moments when my skills were challenged and I had to put all of my effort into achieving something that I wouldn't typically dare to do. After my mother had passed, I entered a fitness competition that required six months of disciplined dieting and rigorous physical training. Sounds difficult, I know, but it was an incredible experience to see my body transform. In the end, I literally stood in front of an audience that applauded my efforts. I didn't do it so I could fit into a tiny bathing suit or claim some kind of medal. I did it for the incomparable thrill of accomplishment, particularly after I had endured such personal hardship. There is a feeling of personal empowerment that occurs when, against all odds, you achieve what you set out to do. In the end, it feels even better than you imagined.

Why is this so important in the realm of loss?

There's a feeling of total satisfaction when you master a personal goal, when your challenges are met and you prevail. This feeling is especially gratifying after you may have felt as though you lost some control in your life, or you've experienced an emotional rut. When you take on a goal that you're determined to achieve, you enter into a zone of new energy, new thought, and new action — all of which you, and only you, will control. No one can take this goal from you if you choose to achieve it.

Some time ago, I quit my nine-to-five office job so I could dedicate my time and energy to writing this book. I set a goal and I took the necessary steps to get there. There were times in my journey when I questioned my decision to leave a 'secure' job and wondered if the path I chose was the right one. Then I refocused. I would think back to the goals that I had set for myself and how desperately I wanted to reach readers like you. I was so determined to achieve my goals that I did not allow distractive thoughts to get in the way of my achievements. I made sure that my goal was strictly dependent on me – and me only.

Likewise, during your own process of goal-setting, be careful not to set goals that rely on other people, or those where your achievements are tied to someone else's actions. You need to make sure it's all about you, and that this goal is under your exclusive control. You might have ambitions to travel the world with your husband, or to take your kids to Disneyland; however, these are not the goals that pertain to this chapter in your life. Those goals may or may not happen, depending on a number of external factors. You need the goal you choose today to be exclusively dependent on you and your will power. This way it is 100% within your power to realize your goal.

Next, ensure you set challenges that are in balance with your own personal skill sets. For example, don't set out to be an astronaut or a Broadway actress, if you don't have training for these things. Be realistic about your goals and, if you want to dream big, be willing to take the necessary steps to get there.

So what's your goal and how are you going to achieve it? If you're not sure what your goal should be, look to areas of your life that are lacking. Perhaps it's not as apparent as something like 'losing weight' or 'going back to school'; maybe it's simply a matter of promising some time to yourself every day without any interruptions or distractions. There's no such thing as a goal that is too big or too small, as long as it's something that challenges you and takes effort to achieve.

Staying on track is crucial, particularly at this time in your life. You have recently experienced a loss and though you are learning to cope as time goes on, your Illness is still fairly new. Loss is especially painful for those who thrive in environments that they can control, and thus they find themselves in very unfamiliar territory. When I lost my mother, I recall waking up with feelings of grief and shock for some time. This was not necessarily because of my mother's death, but because it was the first time in my life that I had experienced an event I had no control over. Regardless of which actions I chose to take on a given day, my mother was *still* gone and always would be. There was nothing I could do about any of it. This feeling was foreign to me, especially because I had once managed all areas of my life so well. I hated the feeling that I could not change the outcome. This isn't to say that I expected everything in my life to go as I had hoped or that I had never known anything to be outside of my control; but this was certainly the first time I experienced something absolutely *final* and *permanent*. Unlike other negative experiences, where I may have dealt with lesser misfortunes, I always felt I had the choice to *do* something with those endings. This was the first time that the outcome was absolute and I could do nothing about it.

Does your Illness leave you feeling like you've lost control? And you're desperately seeking to relieve that dreadful feeling?

Mastering a goal, and sticking with it, is important because it gives you back some of the control you've lost. Good intentions aren't good enough. Although your goal may have nothing at all to do with your Illness, it has everything to do with your overall well-being. Setting a goal and sticking to it, allows you to structure your life at a time when organization is lacking. Your goal will allow you to focus on something other than your Illness, and, hopefully, aside from improving the person you are, it will most likely serve as a distraction or a replacement for your Illness. Thus, seeing it as a substitute for such a dramatic, life-altering experience exemplifies why your goal must challenge your skill sets. If it's too easy, it will not serve you as well as a more challenging goal would at this key moment in your life.

What happens if, despite your best efforts, you feel like you have failed in attaining your goal?

Setbacks are inevitable. These events teach us to remain humble but eager. As long as we don't collapse in the face of our setbacks, we will continue on the road to achieving our goals. Once you set a goal, don't plan for obstacles, but when faced with them, don't give up. Instead ask yourself: "How can I move forward in achieving my goal?" Self-blame will do absolutely nothing for you. You need to acknowledge the setback and move forward. The amount of time you spend dwelling on the unexpected impediment will only grow, draining you of valuable energy.

Mastering a goal is also important because of its outcome. When you succeed at achieving something that you set out to do, you experience a sense of pride and triumph.

So where do you start? If you don't know what goal you want (or need) to accomplish at this point in your life, begin by creating a self-awareness board that describes you.

Answer the following questions in your journal to see the big picture. Don't be afraid to repeat answers, this will simply reinforce areas that you need to focus on.

- What are your 'soft' skills?
- What are your 'hard' skills?
- What skills do you admire in other people that you do not possess yourself?
- Who is your idol? Why?
- What challenges you?
- What makes you happy? Why?
- What three things matter to you most?
- What have you always wanted to do, but have never had the time to do?
- What are your shortcomings?
- What are three small goals you'd like to accomplish in three months?
- What are three larger goals you'd like to accomplish in five years?

Remember: Make sure these goals do not require other people, but instead are within your direct control. (ie. Do not list "getting married" or "having children" as goals. Of course, these may be among the wishes you have for the future; but, at this point, the emphasis of the goal-setting should focus on you only).

Once you answered the above questions, you may recognize a number of goals you would like to accomplish – some easier than others. Start with one short-term goal (one that takes three-six months, or even less), and set out to achieve it. Keep in mind the power of your own choice when you set this goal.

First, ask yourself what you want to gain from your goal. Make sure that obtaining your goal is for your own growth and not for someone else's. For example, if your partner has always wanted you to enroll in a cooking class, but you don't have any interest in this, do not make that your goal. You should want to succeed in achieving this goal with or without the affirmation of anyone else.

Setting goals and doing good things for ourselves isn't selfish, it's imperative (particularly as you grow from your Illness). Too often we assume good things should be done for other people, and that being happy means making other people feel good. Though being kind and compassionate to others does play a role in our overall happiness (see Chapter 6), being kind to yourself must happen first. Simply put: you cannot properly care for others until you have taken care of yourself first. In illustrating this point I'd like to use the analogy of an airplane's safety features. In case of emergency, aircrafts are equipped with oxygen masks for passengers. The instructions always ask that you put on your own mask before assisting a child or someone in need next to you. The reason is the same as mine: you cannot care for others fully without caring for yourself first, even in a life or death situation!

The 10 steps to achieving your goal are:

1. Set your goal
2. Ensure your values promote your goal
3. Give the process a start and end date
4. Believe you can accomplish it
6. Visualize your goal
7. Be your #1 Fan
8. Push yourself
9. Change bad habits, promote good ones
10. Surround yourself with good people

Insisting that your values promote your goal simply ensures that you're living through your Higher Self. This means you're setting goals that are good for you and promote happiness for you and others. For example, it shouldn't be a goal to hurt or sabotage someone even if that person has previously hurt you. Ensure your goal is good-hearted and does not seek to bring anyone else ill feelings.

Giving your goal a start and end date sets parameters. Similar to a school assignment or an office project, you are establishing accountability with yourself. Own your time. List all the necessary steps needed to master the goal and set dates beside each sub-item. Tell people who support you about these timelines. For example, if your goal is weight loss, and you have your target weight set for the end of each week, make it known. Take the deadlines you set seriously and don't dismiss it if you fail to meet them. Repercussions might include admitting to people you trust that you've failed in this aspect of goal-setting and determining ways of preventing this from happening again. Make time for your goals, and be sure to prioritize your time. You can even commit this to writing from start to finish.

Believe you can accomplish your goal. Get up each morning, look in the mirror, and challenge yourself with three "mini goals" to be accomplished in the day ahead. These will assist you in obtaining your final goal. Maybe it's telling yourself not to get angry with anyone today and that instead you will focus on maintaining a healthy mindset. Maybe it's more physical: you'll tell yourself that today you will run an extra five minutes on the treadmill. Whatever it is, say it out loud to yourself and believe it. Today, you will do it!

Next, visualize your goal. Put up pictures of your new body, or the trip you want to take. You want to see and feel your results. The pictures that capture your goal shouldn't just be in one place, but in as many areas of your life as possible. In your wallet, in your bedroom, at work, in the car – there's no place your goal cannot be visualized!

Be your own "#1 fan" when pursuing your goal and promise to support yourself throughout the journey. There will be times when you're on track and it will be easy to think positively about yourself, but there will also be times when setbacks occur and you may feel as though you have failed. Regardless of this, be your own friend throughout the process and cheer yourself on. At night, before you go to bed, take a moment to reflect on the three "mini goals" you had set earlier that morning. Did you accomplish each of them? How does it feel to have conquered these three small challenges? Take pride in each step you take to achieving your overall goal.

Push yourself. Understanding that you may not feel up to it, pushing yourself is sometimes imperative to achieving your goals. Don't wait to get motivated by someone or something, take the initiative yourself. If your goal is to find a new job, push yourself to re-write your resume even if you are frustrated at the lack of responses you have gotten. Force yourself to get up, go to the local coffee shop with wireless connection and dedicate several uninterrupted hours – outside of the house – toward the search for a new career. It's difficult to do at times, but you can't always wait until you feel like it. Maintain focus by visualizing the goal's outcome and how great it will make you feel. The notion of self-starting and pushing through your different setbacks is all part of achieving the goal you have set. After all, we *accomplish* our goals; they aren't handed to us.

Change bad habits and encourage new ones that promote your goals. Habits are simply our routine behaviors, whether conscious or unconscious. If our habits do not encourage our own healthy well-being and support those of others, they need to change and be substituted by those that will. Everything from how you treat others to how you treat yourself needs to be considered. Negative behavior and habits that hurt you physically, emotionally, or spiritually will prevent you from obtaining your goals. This includes everything from negative self-talk to any type of substance abuse. Poisoning yourself or your environment will greatly affect your power to aggressively obtain any goal you set for yourself.

Surrounding yourself with good people and a positive environment should be everyone's daily intention. This may mean separating yourself from people you may have outgrown and who no longer have a positive impact on your life. Look around you. Do the people and places that surround you mirror your values? Are the people in your life supportive of your goals, or do they undermine them? Do they promote a healthy, happy lifestyle that can assist you in achieving your goals through positive reinforcement? Is there anyone you need to hide your goals from, because they may feel threatened by them?

Ask yourself these questions and don't be afraid to hear the honest answers. Good or bad, it will greatly affect your quality of life. If any of the answers to the above questions lead you to believe that your current environment is not conducive to supporting your goals, then you need to separate yourself from those particular people or places. Whether it's old friends, family members, a romantic partner, or your place of work, everything and everyone you choose to surround yourself with should be positive. Those who share your values and reinforce your emotional well-being are the people you want to surround yourself with always. How else can you strive to obtain goals when you don't have the proper support system?

Once you have achieved your goal, savor it! Enjoy it! Too many of us go about our lives so quickly knocking ourselves down for the poor decisions we make or the losses we incur. You need to take the time to congratulate yourself not only at the conclusion of meeting your goal, but everyday, when you get up and decide to continue on with the decision to get your life back on track. Smile at the thought that with each passing day, your Illness is one step further behind you.

Each night, when you go to bed and think about the mini-goals you had set earlier that day, you can smile, knowing that they were accomplished by you. Take note of every goal you seek to accomplish and record how each step makes you feel. What are you noticing? Do you suddenly have a journal full of good deeds and accomplishments? Is it becoming easier to do the things you once imagined you never could? Are you beginning to like the new you, and your new-found desire to change your life? It's exciting to see what goals can do to us – especially when they are in black and white, right in front of us. It becomes about more than just the end result, and you will quickly be more grateful for all the steps you've taken to get there.

Tomorrow is a new day in your journey to overcoming your Illness and obtain happiness, but be sure to stop and appreciate that today functioned as a necessary stepping stone toward reaching that ultimate goal. Remember, goals will be just that, "goals", that is until you take action and make them a reality. Rid yourself of the "I could never do that" mentality and start taking action. Thank your Higher Self for giving you today and for giving you the power to set and achieve your goals.

CHAPTER 6

MASTERING THE NOTIONS OF COMPASSION AND FORGIVENESS

Human beings need to live amongst one another. We rely on each other's strengths and expertise to better our own lives. We visit our doctors when we are sick, we go to the dentist when we need our teeth examined, we go to school to learn from our teachers, and we visit our favorite restaurant when we want to taste a specific dish. Simply put, we need one another to live happier, healthier, more fulfilled lives.

Compassion and forgiveness are required for true peace and happiness. They're particularly important in overcoming our Illnesses. They are an attitude and a process that alleviate emotional pain by showing us the world from another perspective. It's the notion of stepping outside your own views, and stepping into the shoes of another. Because we inhibit this earth together we need to show kindness and consideration to one another, despite our differences. The world is made up of a beautiful array of complicated, diverse individuals. When we lack the ability to see the world through different perspectives, and prevent ourselves from feeling compassion, we deprive ourselves of the very things happiness consists of. You cannot be truly happy without being at peace with yourself and those in your life. And you have not been completely healed from your Illness until you are truly happy with your life and your place in it.

In coping with an Illness it may be especially challenging to find the strength needed to forgive and show compassion to others. Perhaps you feel betrayed or deceived, and thus you think it is impossible to find the power to demonstrate reason and strength. I'm not saying it's easy, but finding your inner power can be learned, and with time, it can be strengthened.

Before we get into *why* we need to show compassion and forgiveness, particularly while coping with an Illness, let us first acknowledge what empathy *is* and what it is *not*. Forgiveness can be a contradiction between the rational mind and our emotional well-being. When one side of our mind is telling us to forgive and let go, the other side reminds us of how hurt we are and how angry we should be. This mental tug-of-war is what can prevent us from moving past our Illnesses, leaving us instead to ruminate on our current state of mind. By acknowledging that compassion and forgiveness may be radical departures from your typical way of thinking, you are able to master this thought process and move away from your pain. Tell yourself, "I have been hurt and I acknowledge that, yet in order to be free from this Illness, I need to let go of the anger that is victimizing me."

Forgiving yourself is just as important as forgiving those around you. This test of maturity and self-love accepts that we are not perfect beings and that we do not always show our best and most loving attributes. Even with good intentions or hope for happier outcomes, we can hurt or betray the people closest to us.

Perhaps your Illness is related to coping with the loss of a loved one whom you feel you have hurt and/or betrayed. Many of my clients prolong the suffering process by either failing to recognize their own mistakes or, on the contrary, continually punishing themselves for things they have done in the past. They are unwilling to let go. They fail to acknowledge their imperfections that make them whole. Our experiences allow us to grow and learn. We need to strive daily to live by the values that we believe; however, when we slip (and we all slip sometimes), we need to stop and forgive ourselves. Allow yourself to be human. Understand that what makes a good person whole is his or her ability to make mistakes, take responsibility for them, and learn to walk away from them. Welcome the gift of self-acceptance.

When we do not show compassion to others, and we choose not to forgive ourselves and those who have hurt us, we hold onto a great deal of pain. In fact, by not letting go, we actually amplify our negative feelings. If our perceptions and thoughts are what make us happy, and we are harboring ill thoughts, we are only hurting ourselves. The definition of happiness simply has no room for grudges or anger – regardless of what acts have transpired.

Letting go of anger is liberating. It frees us of what can be both emotionally and physically draining. Holding on to anger cripples us and keeps us in victim mode. Anger tells us that we *deserve* to be upset, as though such feelings are empowering and somehow thrilling. As mentioned in Chapter 3, anger gives us a false sense of power, fueling us with negative emotions. This false sense of power is especially gratifying when we feel betrayed, violated, or deceived – it's our way of screaming back at the world that life isn't fair. We have been hurt and we have an innate human desire to want to be heard.

We have all been hurt by someone else. We drain our energy and magnify our negative feelings by telling everyone we know how hurt we are. We tell anyone who will listen to us what an evil person our perpetrator is for hurting us, and how he or she does not deserve to be happy. It's easy to fall into this trap, and at times, it can seem somewhat gratifying. The problem, however, is that this type of "self-abuse" is ultimately harmful. Similar to a drug that alters the mind but soon wears off, negative talk only lasts so long before the "high" we get from undermining others subsides. Angry rumination is tempting but never satisfying for any significant period of time.

It's important to note that letting go does not necessarily mean forgetting. For example, it's completely acceptable to let go of ill feelings towards someone else, but ask them to leave your physical world. By forgiving, you are not promising to mend the relationship with the person or people who have wronged you. If a husband or friend has betrayed you, you might tell him or her to leave. If an employer has treated you unfairly, you may decide to find alternative employment. If your religious leader defies your values, you can choose to practice your religion in another temple or spiritual place.

By removing people from your own place of inner peace, you are ridding yourself of negative feelings. You forgive them because we are all human and capable of inflicting pain; however, you don't have to keep these people in your life. By being a compassionate person, you do not have to maintain relationships with particular people who may have hurt you. In some cases, to do so would only inflict further pain and suffering. By forgiving but removing yourself from the lives of others, you are simply saying, "I forgive you because you are human and capable of doing wrong; however, I deserve to be happy and this situation no longer makes me so."

We must show compassion and forgiveness always; however, we must be conscious and considerate of whom we allow into our lives as well. Be aware of who deserves your time and who promotes your happiness. Again, this is a liberating lesson after suffering an Illness.

Next, being compassionate and finding forgiveness does not mean accepting a particular action. By acknowledging why you are hurt or angry and choosing to put it aside (whether you decide to maintain a relationship with the person who has wronged you or not) you are not saying that the act is permissible and acceptable. A wrong is a wrong and that can be very clear. By forgiving someone for an ill act, you are only forgiving the person; you are not accepting the act itself.

In some cases, as was the case for me, I needed to forgive someone who is no longer alive in order to move past my Illness. For me, I needed to acknowledge that my mother was not perfect and that there were times in my life when her drinking caused me a great deal of pain. There were many times when I, along with others in my family, suffered because of her alcoholism. It would be difficult to refute the fact that my mother's own Illness - though she conquered it magnificently - had a profound impact on everyone who loved her.

I needed to let go of this pain. I couldn't get past my Illness without accepting my mother as a whole person, and that meant both the good and bad. I have since taken comfort in knowing that it is because of my mother's imperfections that I have grown to be the person I am today. Her disease strengthened me. Above all, it showed me how not to drink.

I forgave my mother, though I'm not sure when exactly. She stopped drinking several years before her passing and I was well into my adult life when it happened. I like to think I forgave her while she was alive, but perhaps it wasn't until she passed that I truly grasped the complexity of life, and just how fragile it is. On that March evening my world changed, and forgiving my mother was the first step in understanding how delicate life is and how important and precious other people truly are.

What does showing compassion and forgiving ourselves and the people in our lives do for us, particularly when we are coping with an Illness?

1. It makes us whole. Human beings are complex creatures who are not perfect and will inevitably make mistakes. We need to embrace those mistakes as part of our journey and choose to learn from them, taking responsibility for our choices and actions.

2. It makes us strong. Compassion and forgiveness restores inner peace allowing us to no longer be victims of the outside world. We need to learn to let go for our own sake.

3. It makes the world a better place. These kinds of attributes are not only contagious but they also promote happier, more peaceful living. Demonstrating kindness to others should be everyone's moral responsibility.

The next obvious question is, "How?" How do I learn to be more compassionate and forgiving while I am hurt and feeling betrayed or deceived? If I am unable to forgive, how do I learn to move on and forgive myself? How do I incorporate these attributes into the recovery process when I'm already so emotionally weak?

The answers to these questions do not come easily and require effort and time. How much time is dependent on your ability to recognize what feelings are holding you back and your willingness to change your view of them. We will touch more on changing your perception of an Illness (in order to forgive it) later in this chapter.

Begin by finding yourself an ally. Find someone that you can confide in and share your story with. This may be a family member, friend, counselor, or coach. Whoever it is, find someone you can talk with (it's important to note I said talk *with*, not talk *to*). We all need someone to comfort us, if not to offer guidance, rather than to simply listen to us. If it's a family member or friend – as opposed to a paid expert – be careful not to drain them in their efforts to be there for you. We do this when we continually speak negatively, whether it's about ourselves or anyone else in our lives. This kind of negativity pushes people away because they can only endure so much. This is not to suggest that we "sugar coat" the facts to make them more palatable, but, we do need to be willing to move on. If you're continually ruminating on negative thoughts, consider talking with a professional as opposed to a friend or family member.

To address what's holding you back from being compassionate and offering forgiveness, you should start by telling your story. You may even want to write it down in your journal before speaking to someone you trust. Release the details of what has happened to you. In discussing your Illness and asking yourself to address different feelings, note who you are angry with and why you have not yet let go. Be honest. Be willing to abstain from self-judgment and ensure that your confidante is not judging you either. This exercise will help you forgive and let go, and it's not a form of punishment. Whom do you need to forgive? And rather than asking yourself whether you *will* choose to forgive this person, ask yourself *when* you will choose to forgive. Be confident in your answer. Start laying out the steps you will take to get there.

In telling your story, focus on your emotions. What are your feelings telling you? Be conscious of all the negative baggage that you are carrying around with you and how it's affecting your own personal well-being. Though you may want to live a happier life, are you truly trying to rid yourself of this excess emotional baggage? Are you making the necessary effort (and, yes, it takes effort) to break free of the emotions that prevent you from moving past your Illness?

The power of forgiveness and compassion comes from within. It's not dependent on other people. Regardless of the popular belief that empathy is about making others happy, finding forgiveness and learning to be compassionate towards others is an action that we choose based on self-love. It is just as much about making others happy (as we should universally want to promote happiness), as it is about wanting to make ourselves happy.

Once you have released the story of your Illness and you have addressed that you need to forgive (and include yourself if applicable), ask what is preventing you from offering empathy. Uncover your feelings of bitterness and blame. Are you not offering forgiveness and compassion because you simply aren't aware of all your negative thoughts, or is it because these thoughts and perceptions are intertwined with feelings of guilt? Perhaps you're angry that your partner has left you, but you feel guilty that you were not the most loving person to be with. Maybe you are upset that your employer let you go; however, you also know you were continually late and taking days off. You punish yourself by thinking about what could have been and telling yourself that the loss is your fault, that it could have been avoided if only you were a different person. This kind of self-punishment makes it difficult to move past an Illness and offer forgiveness. This is mainly because you are likely to dismiss that you are feeling guilty in the first place. You're stuck between two Illnesses. Acknowledge all your anger – which means making note of everything and everyone you are angry at – and this will help you learn to let go.

Adopt a new perspective and learn to look at the Illness and those involved from a different point of view. Reframe your Illness and those involved (including you) and you will learn to see life in a different light.

In understanding our own suffering, we begin to sympathize and appreciate the suffering of others. It's the notion that we are all human and that our Illnesses are universal, exempting no one. Rather than spending excess time dealing with negative emotions, focus your energy on a better you. Try to consciously change your perspective of the situation. See yourself as owning the situation, as opposed to being victimized by it. My mother was not perfect, perhaps your business partner has betrayed you, or your employer has let you go. Whatever your Illness is, take the time to stand in the other person's shoes. What is going on in their life? What pain or suffering could they be feeling? View the situation as a learning process versus some kind of confirmation that we deserve our respective Illnesses. Recognize that you can become a better person when you love yourself enough to forgive and let go. It's a wonderful, freeing place to be.

Make it a commitment to forgive and offer compassion. This duty to one's self can start the moment you get up in the morning. Rather than dwelling on the negative, learn to say thank you. Even if it's forced at first, get up tomorrow and say thank you for something. Maybe it's your health, maybe it's your friends or family, or maybe it's something as simple as a sunny morning. Say thank you. Remain humble and thankful regardless of the world's imperfections.

Make it a moral responsibility to give back even if it's in the form of simple courtesy. Be conscious of holding doors open for people, or smiling at a neighbor from down the street. It's amazing how uplifting it can be to perform small, effortless tasks like these and to watch how they can completely change your day. It's our ability to connect with others that we often forget. If we are all humans who suffer Illnesses and want to be happy, why do we often forget to do things that make someone else happy? The fact is we all suffer from Illnesses, and you never know when someone's day is worse than your own. Maybe while you are suffering from job loss, someone next to you on the bus is plagued with the reality that her son is dying of cancer. Everyone has a story. We all suffer from Illnesses. No one is exempt.

Ask for help from within. Learn to pray. Connect with your Higher Self often and ask for strength to forgive and become a more compassionate person. Sit quietly and reflect. This does not have to be a religious experience; anyone can connect with their Higher Self. See yourself at peace with the world and everyone in it. Breathe. Ask yourself, "What would life be like if I forgave this person?" Experience the freeing sensation. Practice this kind of self-talk and meditation regularly. Learn to connect this peaceful feeling with learning to forgive and releasing negative emotions.

Forgiveness and compassion are often very difficult; however, when you master the ability to exercise them, you will never be a victim to life's struggles again. We never have to accept someone else's actions, and our forgiveness does not mean our acceptance of a wrong someone has committed against us. We simply need to forgive, and we need to learn to be compassionate because we are human. All of this is part of our own personal growth. Being at peace with people on this earth benefits us individually; it is for our own happiness. If it makes someone else happy as well, then that is an added benefit. We forgive for ourselves first.

Through our personal suffering and our ability to embrace forgiveness, we triumph over the troubles that plague us. Welcome self-love and make it a moral responsibility to promote goodwill. Learn that forgiveness is necessary in living well and that this is part of the process of healing from our Illnesses.

CHAPTER 7

LOVING YOURSELF OUTSIDE OF THE EVENT OR CIRCUMSTANCE

Self-love is like the air that you breathe when it comes to overcoming your Illness: it's absolutely necessary. It's not narcissistic to love yourself; on the contrary, self-love is altruistic because it means you're giving the best possible you to the universe.

Do you love yourself?

Ask yourself, do you talk about yourself the way you do your best friend? Do you reassure yourself and speak highly of your strengths the way you would of those dearest to you? Do you respect yourself the way you do your friends or family members?

I'll give you an example. My best friend is beautiful, kind, and intelligent. She is someone I consider family, and someone for whom I would drop everything if she needed me.

She exudes grace and class effortlessly. I trust her with my deepest secrets, and she never judges me. No matter what she puts on in the morning, she looks wonderful every day. Though she can make someone feel like they are the most important person in a crowd, she's the one, in my opinion, who never goes unnoticed.

Does this sound like your best friend, too?

If I were to appraise myself, on the other hand, I would find it much more difficult. I'm hard on myself when I think I have failed at something, whether it's related to work, relationships, or my fitness regimen. How many people have gotten up in the morning and said, "I look old…or I hate the way I look…I'm overweight." When was the last time you got up and said, "Wow, I look good!"

Do you ever go out with your best friend and tell her she looks fat? Do you tell her you hate her nose? If she tells you that she had a bad day at work last week, do you tell her that it was likely her fault that this happened?

You don't even have to answer these questions, because if it's your dearest friend you are thinking about, the answers are undoubtedly "no." We are all very quick to talk negatively to ourselves (especially when dealing with an Illness), but we would never do so to our closest friends. Is it because everyone's friends really are that pretty or smart? Do our friends never fail at work or in their relationships? Of course they do. Then why don't we belittle our friends the way we do ourselves?

The answer is simple: You're not *choosing* to stop the negative talk with yourself the way you do with those closest to you. You're not *choosing* to see the best in yourself, the way you do with your friends. You're not *choosing* your self-talk; instead, you are allowing your self-talk to choose you. The negative talk can be especially common when dealing with an Illness, a time when positive self-assurance is, in fact, critical.

Similar to the way you choose not to tell your friend you don't like her new outfit, or how you choose to see her strengths when she ends her relationship, you need to learn to make those choices for yourself as well. Before you speak to yourself (and we do this constantly throughout the day, whether it's conscious or unconscious), ask yourself, "Would I say this to my best friend?" If your answer is no, then stop. Don't think about it a second longer if it's not worthy of your time or attention. Choose to be good to yourself to heal your Illness.

Encourage positive self-talk. Not only do we want to stop putting ourselves down, but we should be promoting positive self-talk and encouragement as well. In coping with an Illness, *positive* self-talk should be a priority daily. Just as we would to those closest to us, be sure to praise yourself when you feel it's deserved. Whether it's being proud about how you handled a stressful situation at work, or that you stayed an extra 10 minutes at the gym today, smile at your achievements and recognize them. Don't see them as expectations met, but rather as successes belonging to you.

Positive self-talk is most easily done when you can separate "interpretation" from "facts." We often blur the distinction between the two when we are dealing with an Illness. It's easy to tell yourself you are not pretty enough, or thin enough, but this is an interpretation based solely on your judgment. Is it the case that everyone would agree with you? Is it an *absolute* statement? No, it's not! You're simply comparing yourself to what you see as "perfection", an objective that is unequivocally unreachable. Human beings aren't perfect, that's a fact.

Negative self-talk can be a self-sustaining cycle. Often unaware of its patterns, we promote negative thoughts that can immobilize us, and leave us feeling worthless and insignificant. One thought leads to another and in a matter of minutes we've envisioned a future of hopelessness and despair. I recall even as a young child watching my mother's drinking and how I allowed it to feed my negative thinking. At times her disease made me so angry I would shatter dishes or bang walls just to be heard. When she was at her lowest, I would convince myself that perhaps my family was just cursed, that it would never get better, and that I would hide this secret from everyone for the rest of my life. A mission that I later learned was not only destructive to my healing, but completely exhausting.

Loving yourself outside of your Illness illustrates how people should not be able to destroy us emotionally. People will affect your happiness and you will affect theirs; however, *affect* doesn't mean *determine*. Only you can determine and choose to be happy. And in order to be happy, you need to love yourself first. You want to like the person you are. You should be familiar with your strengths and take pride in your accomplishments. Loving yourself allows you to be less vulnerable to other people's opinions and less dependent on their praise and acknowledgment to make you happy.

Do you have self-love? To find out, complete the following exercise in your journal.

List 5 things you like about yourself
List 5 things you dislike about yourself
List 5 things you like about a friend/ partner

Recognize the differences and similarities in your answers. What do you notice? The point of the exercise is for you to get to know yourself a bit better while simultaneously recognizing your insecurities and desires. Take time to answer these questions and try to think outside the box with your answers. Make sure the things you like about yourself are things that make you smile. No doubt there are a number of qualities you've never even given yourself credit for. Search for them.

Perhaps your list of your own 'likes' pertains strictly to how you make other people feel, or what you give back to your community, family, or partner. Maybe everything you like about yourself is connected to other people or your relationships with them. Self-love means loving yourself outside of other people as well. It means loving your life and wanting the best for it. If your community, family, or partner were taken away from you, how would your answers change?

Next, examine your dislikes. Ask yourself: Why are these things important to me? Should they be? Do they add value to my life? Are they superficial or genuine in nature? What do you need to work on and when do you plan to start?

When writing both lists – your likes and dislikes – consider which list is easier to compose. Did you have to really ponder your 'likes' while you were quick to identify your 'dislikes'? As you write in your journal you will likely take note of how hard you are on yourself, and how much praise you give to others in your life. If possible, do this exercise with a close friend or family member. Watch how someone else views you in comparison to how you view yourself.

Finally, consider your last list. The list that describes the top five things you like about your partner or friend. Are those qualities or characteristics the same as your own list of 'likes'? Again, this goes back to my description of my best friend, and how I feel she lights up a room. I want you to start seeing yourself the way you view those closest to you. There are countless people who think you are wonderful: learn to agree with them and take the time to appreciate what they see in you.

Next, I want to examine self-respect as it is so highly connected to self-love. One simply cannot exist without the other. No one can give you self-respect and no one can take it away without your conscious or unconscious consent. Self-respect begins with you – with the way you choose to think and the way you choose to behave. It means accepting you for you and acknowledging your experiences, both good and bad, as part of your make-up. Don't let your ex-employer, your former spouse or partner, or any other person or circumstance, take your happiness from you. It belongs to you and only you can relinquish it.

What happens if I don't like myself, or respect my own existence?

Self-love will determine your happiness. Not only will it affect your moods and behaviors, but it will have a direct impact on how others treat you as well. People cannot value others who don't value themselves. When you don't love yourself, it shows. Lacking self-worth tells the world, "I don't deserve to be happy, and I need other people's assurance to feel good about myself." Consequently, you will constantly be vulnerable to others' opinions of you. Other people will determine your self-worth, because you won't determine your own. People's judgments or assumptions about you will matter far more than they should, because you won't value yourself outside of their opinions. It's not love if you are asking someone else to give your life significance.

Be careful that your Illness does not prevent you from loving yourself or respecting yourself. I've worked with many people who, when dealing with an Illness, feel so low that they are not only aware of their lack of self-love, they also feed the cycle.

When my mother was at her weakest, and she allowed drinking to take over her life, she did not love herself enough to separate herself from her Illness. She allowed it to become a part of herself (and consequently, a part of the entire family). My mother's Illness and her lack of self-respect functioned as a poisonous cycle, with one problem feeding the other one. Though she finally triumphed over her Illness, this wasn't possible until she chose to love herself above all else.

Ultimately, in my mother's case she did eventually choose to see her Illness as something she could separate herself from. This was how she finally gained control over her disease. As any addict can attest, this is an incredible feat and one that I am so proud she was able to accomplish. My mother learned from conquering her own Illness that when you treat yourself kindly and positively, you learn to love and respect yourself. You accept your past but you don't dwell on it. Though you love the people in your life, it's not their love for you that allows you to value your own existence. You love yourself outside of their praise or criticism. You're at peace with yourself and you can acknowledge that, while you may not be able to choose everything that happens to you (since we don't typically choose our Illnesses), you can certainly choose how you will react.

Tell yourself:

- I am my own person
- I choose to see my body and my physical appearance simply as extensions of me, not as things that define who I am
- I choose to value my existence outside of other people's opinions
- I choose to acknowledge that everyone will hold opinions, but I understand that opinions are not facts
- I make mistakes and choose to learn from them
- I choose to take responsibility for my decisions and my actions
- I choose to see myself as a complex human being who is constantly striving to be a good person, but who will not sacrifice her/his own happiness for the sake of someone else's opinions.

Let me be clear in that I am not suggesting that when we undergo loss, we are indifferent or that we don't feel pain; I'm quite familiar with the contrary. That said, because we are not exempt from Illnesses (and we will continue to experience them for the rest of our lives), we need to love ourselves outside of everything around us, whether that be the people in our lives, our job titles, or our financial status. All of these can change suddenly; therefore, our becoming dependent on any of them allows them to determine our happiness, potentially leaving us in a constant state of fear and anxiety.

When you don't love yourself, you will often seek love (or what we deem to be love) elsewhere. It is human nature to want to feel connected to other people, and often when we don't respect ourselves we will go to desperate means to fill this void. Many will seek out casual flings and sex in order to find fulfillment. Others will abuse drugs or alcohol trying to numb pain and bring happiness. When you don't love yourself, and you're chasing the dream of being happy, it can be a scary cycle of self-abuse. This vicious cycle will inevitably yield results that are consistent with our sense of worthlessness. We base our actions on our beliefs, and when you believe you're not worthy of something like love or respect, you are likely to attract loveless and disrespectful people into your life.

Imagine life without your relationships, your job, your bank account, and your social status. Are you happy with who you are outside of all this? Would you love yourself the way you do your best friend? Does your self-love depend on these circumstances that can be taken from you?

Loving yourself means appreciating the good that you can bring to yourself every day. Stop any negative self-talk, and begin to talk to yourself the way you would a dear friend. Start the day off tomorrow by getting out of bed and acknowledging what you will bring to the day, and *not* what the day will bring to you. How will you choose to create your day, versus waiting to see what the day has in store for you?

How do you do this? Start with self-affirmation speeches or what I call, "I am" speeches.

Stand in front of the mirror, look yourself in the eye and try an "I am" speech out loud by yourself. "I am" speeches should refer to the kind of person you want to be, or the kinds of things you want to see happen on a given day. For example, "*I am* going to give a good presentation at work today." "*I am* going to be confident tonight at the party. "*I am* going to make a good impression at the job interview today".

Despite the fact that you're speaking about something that hasn't yet taken place, be sure to verbalize it with conviction. Say each statement to yourself, and repeat it 10 consecutive times. Be sure to phrase your statement without any negatives. For example, "*I am not* going to be angry today", should be "*I am* going to be happy today."

Other "I am" speeches include:

- I am going to work out today
- I am going to do well on my exam today
- I am going to make peace with my husband today
- I am going to speak up in class today

Perhaps your "I am" speech is not necessarily directed toward an action, but rather is connected to a feeling or emotional state. These types of "I am" speeches are great, too, and are just as influential as those connected to an action. Here are some examples:

- I am going to trust myself today
- I am going to laugh a lot today
- I am going to smile regularly today
- I am going to speak encouragingly today
- I am going to relax today

The reason "I am" speeches are so powerful is that they train your mind to visualize a goal. Similar to hypnosis, where someone can change a habit by believing and wanting for it to happen, an "I am" speech is founded on the idea that you can will something into existence. You're telling yourself something that you not only believe can happen, but that you strongly desire for it to happen as well. You want to be confident in today's seminar, and though you know you're nervous, you can imagine being calm and collected when you speak. This type of self-talk, along with visualization is a great tool for positive thinking. It not only starts your day off with a sense of purpose, allowing you to feel good and productive, it actually sends out a positive message about you to the world.

What is your "I am" speech going to say? What will you say to yourself tomorrow 10 times in front of the mirror? What message do you want to confirm within yourself and send out to the rest of the universe? It's in your hands.

Self-talk is essentially the gate-keeper to our thoughts. It tells our mind what thoughts can stay and which ones should leave. When we choose to speak kindly and positively to ourselves, we encourage good thoughts and promote happiness and good feelings. When we speak negatively to ourselves, we inevitably think negative thoughts, and subsequently feel unhappy.

Did you realize the amount of power you had over your thoughts, and therefore your own happiness, in reciting an "I am" speech? Are you owning your thoughts or letting them own you?

Consider the following exercise. In your journal, jot down all of your thoughts pertaining to your Illness. Don't over-think your list, instead simply write what you feel. Your list may reveal conflicting feelings, and that's okay. We're complicated beings and rarely do we experience anything with black and white clarity. It's more typical to love *and* hate someone than it is to like someone unequivocally every day.

Create your list. Analyze your list. What does it tell you about your thoughts? Recognize how much negativity you allow into your mind. If you have more negative thoughts on your list than you do positive ones, understand that you're choosing to think these thoughts. We all choose how we see the world. This doesn't mean that we should be naïve and always see things as though they're good when they're not. That said, choosing to see something as either good or bad, and deciding whether it's worthy of your thoughts for an extended period of time, is entirely up to you. You are the gatekeeper to your own thoughts and therefore, your own happiness.

Loving yourself and respecting the life you lead means valuing everything that you put into your mind and body. It means surrounding yourself with people and an environment that will be kind to you, and allow you to grow. Consider every element in your life as an ingredient to your overall happiness. Whether it's your thoughts, the food you eat, the people you surround yourself with or the place you choose to live, everything says something about how much you love the person you are, and the respect you have for yourself as a human being.

CHAPTER 8

UNDERSTANDING YOUR ILLNESS AND KNOWING WHAT IT HAS DONE FOR YOU POSITIVELY

Though it's difficult to imagine seeing anything positive associated with your Illness, the passing of time will show you how to do this. Our deepest sorrows teach us pain; however, it's only when we're at our lowest that we truly appreciate happiness. Experiences make us feel the depth of our emotions. They reveal our willingness to learn.

When I first lost my mother, I had a choice. I could curl up in resentment, negativity, and fear, or I could take this life-altering experience and turn it into something that would help me grow. I chose to have this life event impact me in a positive way.

When we experience an Illness, it's easy to feel sorry for ourselves and wallow in negative thoughts or emotions. We look at life as though it's not fair, and question how we arrived at our current situation. We trace our steps, and find ourselves thinking about how we could have changed things. We think that, somehow, we could have prevented the state we find ourselves in today. "If I were more compassionate, maybe he wouldn't have left me." "If I had worked longer hours, maybe my employer wouldn't have let me go." "If I were more honest, maybe we'd still be friends."

Though the answers to these propositions may have affected your current state, the fact of the matter is, life often unfolds in ways we do not plan. Whether it was through your own lack of effort, someone else's, or it was simply a matter of life's unpredictability, there was a fork in the road and you're now in a different place. The feelings and emotions that accompany this journey will undoubtedly make you uncomfortable, sad, angry or anxious; however, understanding that this new place is just that – a "new place" – takes the sting out of the lessons that can be learned if we so choose.

In trying to seek the positive aspects of any life-altering experience, or Illness, it's important to note life's detours. Many of us grow up with the notion that our lives will unfold in a very predictable manner. At a young age, girls dream about looking like princesses on their wedding day, living in a beautiful home, and having children they can grow old with. Boys envision making the football team, graduating from college, and earning a six-figure income. Obviously, these are stereotypes; however, the point is not in the particulars of our childhood dreams, but that we all have (or have had) very clear visions of how our lives would unfold. The notion that life has detours shows us that though we can dream, we are not exempt from life's harsh realities. People do not plan for divorce, heartbreak, terminal sicknesses, unexpected deaths, or the inability to have children. We tend to close our eyes to these realties despite their rates of incidence. We would rather plan our lives as though we are exempt from painful experiences, and assume that it's in fact possible to live a fairy-tale life.

Seeing life as having detours (before they actually happen) teaches us that, though we can plan and hope for certain things in our lives, we should be looking through a wider-angle lens. Rather than assuming there is only one road ahead, consider that there are always several paths, and that, although all roads are different, each can take us forward if we allow it to.

Everyone's number one objective in life is to be happy. Whether this means holding a lavish wedding one day, or having a certain number of children, or whether it relates to the money we would like to earn, or the prestige we hope to have, our ultimate goal remains the same: to achieve happiness. That said, rather than assuming there's only one path to living happily, delight in the fact that there are several! Though your journey may steer you left or right, it will never be a dead-end, but rather a matter of mere detours, as long as you see all the roads.

What roads lie ahead of you? What has your Illness taught you? In what ways have you grown?

Perhaps it has taught you that life is short or unpredictable. Maybe it has taught you that you were in an unhealthy relationship and you need to seek more stable companionship. Perhaps your learning is related to health, love, or finance.

In your journal, list 10 things you have learned from your Illness. Be honest and remember that only you will see it.

To exemplify the types of lessons one might learn through their Illness, consider the list shown below. This is the list I created after losing my mother. Notice that many of my lessons are broad in scope, and that, for the most part, they pertain to leading a fuller and more balanced lifestyle. In creating your list, ensure that at least half of your lessons pertain to what you want out of life as a result of your Illness.

After losing my mother, I learned that:

- Life is short and we most likely do not know when our last day on earth will be (or anyone else's either)
- Life is unpredictable and we cannot always plan for what will happen
- Life is not always fair and we are not exempt from ill experiences
- I want to value each day as though it were my last and never assume that there is another day to undo the wrongs I may have created today
- I want to help people cope with loss, as I have learned from my own

- I want to bring peace to the lives of others because I know what it is like to suffer
- I want to take pride in my work because it reflects who I am
- I want to feed my body with good foods so I can live a long and healthy life
- I want to feed my soul with good energy and relaxing activities to ensure a healthy, balanced lifestyle
- I want to love and respect myself to my very core because as long as I am a living, breathing entity, I have that responsibility to myself, those around me, and the world as a whole.

Listing what you've learned from your Illness can be a difficult task; some may argue that it's an impossible one, depending on what the experience entails. I disagree. Though it's not always easy, and it may take several attempts, we can always learn from our experiences if we choose to do so.

Once you have listed your lessons, ask yourself what's next. As a result of your Illness, what possibilities or opportunities lie ahead of you?

As a result of my Illness, my circumstances may have changed, but how can I be better?

1. What do I have more time to do now?
   - Relax/ time to yourself
   - Fitness
   - Dating
   - Creative projects

2. Is there something I have always wanted to do that I could not do before?
   - School
   - Travel

3. What are the types of people I want to align myself with who will assist me with my new goals?
   - Coaches
   - Positive thinkers
   - People who have experienced the same circumstances (grievance counselors, advisors and related workshops)

4. Is there anyone I need to distance myself from?
- Those who bring me down emotionally
- Those who do not share my values
- Those who do not support my goals

5. What are my six-month, one-year, and five-year plans?

To learn from something, and to see it as something that can affect you positively, means choosing to perceive any situation (good or bad) as an experience that plays a part in your growth. Just as we need to burn our hands as children in order to learn not to touch the stove, regardless of how many times we are told it will hurt, we need to experience lows in our lives to grow as human beings.

It may be the case that you were seriously betrayed, and your Illness is entangled in feelings of not only pain, but also extreme anger and resentment. Betrayal is a difficult situation in that in centers on your values and likely the values you presumed that you shared with someone else. Learning from betrayal starts with separating yourself from the event (as explained in Chapter 2), and choosing to see the injustices of the world as part of the complexities that make up this universe (we will discuss life's inconsistencies later in this chapter). Don't beat yourself up and ruminate about how and why it all happened. Instead, choose to focus on you. Focus on your thoughts and your current emotional state. What are you choosing to think about? (Refer back to the last assignment in Chapter 7) Understand that your feelings can be influenced by your thoughts. How can you change your thoughts and consequently your feelings?

You can't change what has already happened; however, you can choose how you will react, and what thoughts you will entertain in a given situation. Feelings are subject to perception. Choose to perceive any situation, even a betrayal, as a circumstance that you will grow from. Call on your greatest strengths to guide you away from feelings of despair.

Understanding that we all have the ability to learn from our Illnesses is important in the healing process. When we learn from our Illness, we automatically welcome positive healing powers. We are shifting our thoughts away from a negative and detrimental state to a positive and helpful one. Choosing to learn from every situation welcomes good thoughts, and consequently positive emotions and behaviors.

Learning to be a survivor is an exhilarating stage all in itself. My father epitomized this, and he was inspiring to learn from. When we first lost my mother, my father was broken. He was visibly uncomfortable when he left the house for extended periods at a time, even if he was with family. He could not be in one place for very long, instead seeking quietude and solace most of the time. I recall all of us visiting my eldest sister's house shortly after my mother's passing to have lunch as a family. Things seemed to be going fine, when suddenly my father asked when we would be leaving. Clearly uncomfortable, my father asked if we could wrap things up and let him go home.

After about six months, my father's healing became more and more noticeable. He went to social dances and community events. He enrolled in grief counseling, and it was then that he began new relationships. It was incredible to watch someone who had every reason to be angry at the world stand up and say, "I choose to live!" He learned to see choices from his Illness. He chose to uphold the spirit of life over death. His ability to step back into life was breath-taking, I remember thinking to myself that I didn't even want to mention it or congratulate him for fear that he might notice it and stop.

Understanding that life and the people in it are complicated and unpredictable is a lesson that should not be dismissed as obvious. Truly embracing this concept is difficult to do, especially when it means we may get hurt in the process. Sometimes we simply need to take pleasure in knowing that whatever it is we are dealing with right now will pass. Life is full of complex processes, and understanding this equips us for its turbulence.

It's important to accept that life doesn't always make sense and not everything has an answer. Sometimes we simply have to stop, breathe and accept life as it is without desperately trying to fix it or the people in it. Understand that, just as you are a complex, sometimes contradictory, person – so is everyone else. We should therefore not be surprised when these complexities and inconsistencies clash. It is inevitable. And at times, the result is pain.

My mother's alcoholism and her sudden death are instances that prompted me to consider the complexity of life. On one hand I had a mother who I know loved me and wanted only good things for me. On the other hand, her drinking caused me so much pain and suffering. When she died, it felt like the universe had stolen my mother from me.

Life is not always fair and people can be unpredictable. When we finally accept that life does not always make sense, we have made a giant leap in the healing (and living) process. Sometimes all you need to cope with a particular situation is the knowledge that you don't have to fix it. But just because you can't fix it doesn't mean you can't handle it.

Learning to calm yourself, especially in dealing with your Illness, is paramount in everyday living. Learn what soothes you. When you recognize the ability we all have to calm ourselves, it can be a powerful tool in every aspect of your life. When you find yourself thinking negative thoughts or feeling negative emotions, stop yourself immediately. Remove yourself from the situation. Try to speak as few words as possible and concentrate on the inner you. Assure yourself that you will handle this situation without asking yourself how. Confidently tell yourself that this moment will pass and that you have the choice to be calm. Concentrate on your breathing.

This exercise can be done everywhere. Whether you're coping with your Illness, frustrated at work, or arguing with your partner, learning to calm yourself in any situation brings peace to you and those around you. It is a wonderful ability that we all have. Practice it.

Learning from your experiences is exciting because rather than dwelling on the past we are focusing on the moment. We are taking an event or circumstance and making it work for us instead of being victimized by it. Assuming you have taken the necessary time to grieve and feel different emotions (without ruminating), choosing to grow is an empowering and thrilling process.

You will be rewarded abundantly by learning from your Illness, despite the pain you have felt, or are currently feeling. Don't discount the things right in front of you that may seem obvious, or the small things that can help make the next chapter in your life happier and more fulfilling. We learn new things every day; it is simply a matter of choosing to recognize them and allowing ourselves to grow from them.

CHAPTER 9

THE FORMULA FOR HAPPINESS

Despite the fact we have witnessed all sorts of crises, our universal goal as human beings is to be happy. Whether you believe that your happiness can be achieved through financial success, a love relationship, or a prestigious lifestyle, the fact that you want to be happy is an inherent part of human nature.

The keys to welcoming happiness into your life are three-fold. First, understand that everyone deserves to be happy, including you. Second, understand that happiness is a choice regarding our reactions to different circumstances. And finally, appreciate that being happy means accepting a life with some degree of pain and understanding that you cannot truly be happy without experiencing some sadness first.

Unfortunately, we often do not make conscious efforts to invite happiness into our lives. Because many of us connect our happiness with external factors, we tend to associate contentment with the ability to acquire and hold onto these things. For example, if we cannot keep a job or stay in a marriage, these so-called "failures" can make us think we don't deserve to be happy. Simply put, happiness can seem like a "prize" or a "reward" for people who have succeeded in different areas of life. In this case, being successful means "sticking it out" and not quitting.

This rationale is obviously flawed. Happiness comes from the inside out, and thus does not hinge on our successes or failures unless we allow it to. (Note: Divorce, job loss or any other kind of unexpected circumstance is only a "failure" if you deem it as such). Because being happy is an inherent virtue, we are all worthy of this state of being. The good news is that it's a "gift" for the taking for whoever wants it, with no strings attached!

Right after my mother's passing, my eldest sister went through an extended period of guilt where she consciously refused herself happiness. Because she was living in a different province and completing a university degree when my mother died, she felt guilty that she was not there for her final days. This was compounded by the fact that three days prior to my mother's death, she did not reach out to speak with my mother on her 59th birthday. My sister felt as though she should have done things differently, and because she did not, she somehow needed to punish herself.

What my sister initially failed to realize was that her actions could not have prevented or in any way changed the fate of my mother on that day in March. Whether she was there in the house when it happened, or whether she had spoken with my mother days before, my mother's death was inevitable and was in no way connected to my sister's actions or lack thereof. Rather than viewing the situation as a matter of bad timing, she internalized it and punished herself by stripping herself of the right to be happy.

These thought patterns are common when dealing with an Illness. It's easy to blame yourself for just about anything, and to punish yourself after the fact for not doing something. We are quick to assume that we do not deserve to be happy when we feel we should have handled things differently. This is when it's imperative to understand that although some situations are not within our control, we can control our reactions to them. My sister could not have controlled the fact that she would be halfway across the country when my mother passed away. The only part of this scenario that she could control was how she would deal with it. And rather than beating herself up, she needed to allow herself the human right to be happy, relieving herself of any unwarranted regrets associated with my mother's inevitable passing. Like everyone, my sister deserved to he happy.

Next, understand that happiness is a choice. You can be happy right now if you choose to. You need to start with the decision to be happy and except that you don't need money, a fabulous body, or a relationship in order to obtain it. Happiness starts from the inside, and begins with you allowing it to prosper.

Choosing happiness is about mastering your thought process. Though I have stated this several times throughout the course of this book, it is worth mentioning again. Because your feelings are extensions of your thoughts, monitoring what you think about will ultimately change your feelings and, essentially, your well-being. For example, let's say you're making a lifestyle change and you want to go to the gym daily but you perceive it to be too difficult or time-consuming. You will likely feel so overwhelmed that you won't make the effort. However, if you choose to change your thought process and think of the workouts as an opportunity to regain a healthy body, exercise will suddenly become exciting and you will regard the gym as a place of personal rejuvenation.

To begin re-programming your thought process, you may have to begin by *pretending* that you think happy thoughts regularly. For example, have you ever known someone who always seemed to be in a good mood? Someone that you look to and say to yourself, "Wow, I wish I was more like that. Nothing seems to bother that person!" When re-programming your thoughts, you need to assume the role of the person you wish to be – a person who thinks positively by nature. Think of it as a play for which you have to "get into character."

Be very conscious of your mind and what you are thinking about. If you find you are feeling down but don't know why, look at the thoughts you let linger in your mind. As soon as you notice any negative feelings, change your thinking immediately. Tell yourself that you will only give attention to positive thoughts – and commit to this. Make it a goal to think positively, even if it means acting out of character. You will find that after time, thinking positively no longer feels like "role playing" but will come as second nature.

Next, examine your perceptions and beliefs about the world and your place in it. What do you see? How do you feel? Most people who claim to be unhappy, often because of a major life experience, have not yet made the connection between their beliefs or perceptions of the world and the way they are currently feeling.

To illustrate this point, think back to when you were a child. Recall when life seemed simple and carefree. Granted, you didn't have the mortgage, children, or financial strains that you may have now, but you were still a human being with a belief system as to how the world worked. You likely dreamt about what you would be when you grew up, and the younger you were, the larger and bolder your dreams. When you were five, maybe you wanted to be the next president, a professional athlete, or the doctor who would find a cure for cancer. The younger we are, the more capable we are of determining our own happiness and presuming that all things are possible. As a child, you determined your own happiness and belief system, and you continued to do so until the rest of the world's belief system got to you.

Beliefs are simply our perceptions of how life *should* unfold. From the moment we are born until the day we die, the people and events that make up our existence will help shape our belief system. Whether it's how we view identity, politics, religion, love, work, parenting, or what it means to be happy, our perceptions are based largely on our subconscious mind and the beliefs that were handed to us as we grew up.

Rather than maintaining that care-free attitude that you had as a child – when you believed everything was possible and happiness was yours for the taking – we adopt the belief systems of those people who surround us as we get older, which can make happiness seem harder to acquire. We are often taught that when we lose something – whether it's a relationship, career, money, and so on – we have failed. Consequently, we begin to believe that happiness means having all of this, and that when even one component of this 'happiness formula' is lost, we have been unsuccessful in at least one aspect of our lives. Our environment and the people around us have been instrumental in determining our belief systems. Unfortunately, many of the beliefs we hold as adults are not conducive to living happily.

How am I capable of happiness if I lost my job and my belief system tells me that losing my job means I am a failure? What happened to the magical world I lived in when I was a child, a world where this kind of loss would have meant something better was just around the corner?

Simply put, we are born into the magical world of our own innate perceptions – a world that is simple and carefree, and it's because of our environment that we begin to take on the belief systems that will essentially determine how profound our Illnesses are. And it's those beliefs that will affect how we react and ultimately recover from our losses.

To exemplify this point, consider the scenario where a wife and husband with three children seek divorce after 12 years of marriage. For the well-being of everyone involved, the family maintains a healthy friendship whereby the children understand that though their parents are no longer together, they respect each other as human beings and want the best for everyone.

Next, consider a wife and husband who, despite an unhealthy marriage, decide not to split because they feel their children need to grow up in a "traditional" nuclear family. The children grow up watching their parents argue daily, and they grow numb to the disrespect and animosity that fills their home.

In both cases the children enter the world "belief-free". As they grow up they consider what is right and wrong about their environment.

In the first scenario, where the parents split but maintain their friendship, the children are likely to grow up with values that reflect the love, respect and understanding they witnessed despite a divorce. Mom and Dad can enter into future love relationships with new partners and they can rest assured that they have taught their children that love and respect will always remain between them as parents. In essence, happiness is not determined by the marriage, but rather by the value each person has for themselves and everyone else in their lives.

In the second scenario, where the parents remain in an unhealthy marriage, the children may grow up believing that arguments and betrayal are a natural part of marriage, and that hardships (no matter how physically or emotionally draining they may be) are simply part of life. Even if the children are aware that such abuse is not right and they promise that they will never be a part of such relationships, these kids will likely grow up thinking that the importance of staying together outweighed their parents' happiness.

Now consider the following questions: Which set of children are more likely to have a difficult time demonstrating respect within their own marriages? Which set of children are more likely to carry resentment and fear into their own marriages? Which are more likely to wrestle with personal issues pertaining to self-respect or self-identity? Which set of children are more likely to endure sustained feelings of unhappiness? The fact is, deeply held beliefs tend to manifest themselves into reality, and if you believe something to be true you will likely make it come true.

Let me be clear in stating that I don't contend that those who are forced to face hardships as children are destined to live unhappy lives. Obviously, many of these children grow up with more stamina than the rest of us. Countless people – myself included – grew up witnessing a lot of suffering, yet they manage to thrive in life. Many excel because of the hard-won battles they dealt with as children.

That being said, it remains that our belief system is strongly connected to our environment. Even though I learned from my mother's alcoholism that I would never make my children feel as awful as I sometimes did, I also learned that alcoholism is a very complex disease. My belief system taught me compassion and love. At an early age I realized that alcoholism hurts everyone involved, not just the person who is drinking. I believed it could destroy the whole family or, alternatively, it could force them to band together to beat the disease; the choice is up to everyone involved. It is because of my mother's alcoholism that I know what it means to be human, and that even the people who love you the most can bring you to your knees.

Once you understand how your belief system is influenced by your environment, it becomes clearer that your surroundings and the people you allow into your life carry such importance. Our beliefs are directly connected to our willingness to be happy, and yet in most cases, our values and what we perceive to be "the right way of doing things" is actually handed to us. We are not born valuing things. We may have an innate need to be loved, fed, bathed and cared for as infants, but we do not come into the world with cultural, political, and religious values – the views that have a huge impact on our ability to be happy.

I'm not suggesting you should reject or dismiss the beliefs that are handed down to you. Your parents or guardians likely handed down a belief system that they felt strongly about and that they believed would make the world a better place for you. That being said, as generations pass and the world changes, belief systems need to be questioned, too.

Take a look at your belief system. Is it bringing you happiness? Do your values reflect what you believe makes you happy, or what someone else believes will make you happy? When you shed your code of beliefs, what lies underneath? Is it a happier, more relaxed you?

Have a look at the chart on the following page and draw the same one in your journal. Be honest about your answers as you fill in the individual boxes. Note that the questions elicit non-judgmental answers. The point of the exercise is not to assess your beliefs or those of your family or friends, but rather to see how similar and connected your answers to these questions may be. The important thing to keep in mind when completing this exercise is your honesty in expressing your personal beliefs.

	Do you maintain this belief? (Yes/ No)	Does your family (or those closest to you) hold the same belief? (Yes/ No)
Do you believe in a higher power?		
Do you believe in marriage?		
Do you believe in divorce?		
Should the man (and not the woman) in the home be responsible for the main source of income?		
Do you believe it is acceptable to not want children once married? (assuming both husband and wife are capable of conceiving a child)		
Do you believe in abortion?		
Do you believe in same-sex marriage?		
Do you believe in monogamy?		
Are you opposed to recreational drugs?		
Do you believe money has a lot to do with happiness?		

Chances are most of your answers in column A are the same as those in column B. Now that you have completed this exercise, and you understand that your family, partner, and friends have influenced your belief system, is there any answer(s) you would change if you knew no one would judge you for doing so? Perhaps your Illness would not be as painful if your belief system was not so opposed to the way you were feeling.

We have already established that thoughts come before feelings and consequently what you allow into your mind will inevitably affect how you feel. Beliefs, however, encompass them all. First you believe the world "ought to be" a certain way; as a result you think certain thoughts, and in the end, you feel a certain way. In essence, the road to welcoming happiness is much more in your control than you may have originally thought. You're not at the mercy of life and what happens to you – you are simply at the mercy of your perception of it!

Ensure the beliefs and the thoughts you give attention to allow you to be happy. Question values that don't support the bumps that are inevitable in life and that don't allow you to learn and grow as a person. Understand that people are complex beings and that perfection is a relative term.

Finally, in order to truly welcome happiness back into your life after undergoing an Illness, you need to be willing to endure some degree of pain and appreciate that happiness does not exist without sadness. The only way to know what happiness feels like is to know what hurt feels like. Sorrow inevitably strengthens us.

Our losses are like illnesses (or sicknesses) in that they will touch our lives, often unexpectedly, over and over until the day we die. Just like we can anticipate getting sick occasionally throughout our lives, we will experience Illness in the same manner. It's simply part of life. This philosophy reiterates the notion that sorrow is an inherent part of the human experience. As much as we resist it – just as we do the common cold – sadness will weave in and out of our lives continually. No one can live a life without experiencing what I define as an Illness; however, it's because of our losses that we are able to experience happiness. One cannot exist without the other.

Our lowest and most painful moments will teach us to appreciate happiness. The feelings associated with your Illness can teach you compassion, resilience, humility, and forgiveness – all of which are ingredients to living happily.

Consider what history has taught us; recall how our painful experiences have promoted wonderful results. If it weren't for world wars, we would not have the gift of freedom. Surviving cancer pushed Lance Armstrong to win the Tour de France. The horrific acts of 9/11 prompted safer airport security check-points and gave the world the opportunity to join hands to experience the gift of humility together.

We have experienced, and will continue to experience, Illnesses as individuals, countries, and as a whole planet; however, it is because of these Illnesses that we will continue to strive for happiness. It's when we are at our lowest moments that we have learned about our most fascinating attributes. Our Illnesses, and our triumphs over them, are necessary ingredients to the recipe for happiness.

CHAPTER 10

EXERCISING THE MIND, BODY AND SOUL

Exercising the mind, body and soul is the final stage of the healing process. This is central to everyday healthy living. As we encounter Illnesses throughout our lives, it is the balance that we maintain within ourselves that will allow us to grow and recover as human beings.

"Soothing the mind" is a term used to refer to the release of stress and the acquisition of a calm, collected mindset. Most people know how important it is to nourish the body with wholesome foods; however, we do not take as much interest in focusing on the well-being of our minds. Though a healthy body is important (we will discuss this later in this chapter), a healthy mind is what ultimately determines our happiness. If our minds are healthy we always have the ability to overcome our Illness.

Exercising the mind starts by acknowledging that your thoughts matter more than any event or circumstance you may encounter. Simply put, our thoughts outweigh any of our Illnesses. Unfortunately, because we are so emotionally connected to our Illnesses, we tend to believe the opposite. We internalize what "happens to" us, and take little notice of what we spend our time thinking about. Events seem larger than our thoughts, and yet it is our thoughts that give them significance in the first place.

A thought does not affect you until it is given some degree of importance. For example, any event or circumstance – either good or bad – is only significant if you give it sustained attention. You feed any event its importance by giving it thought, and not the reverse.

Next, learn to soothe your mind by recognizing what calms you. We are all different people, and therefore, we are affected by negative stimuli in different ways. This not only pertains to dealing with an Illness but also to coping with everyday life. It's important to be conscious of both. Take note of the things that leave you feeling uneasy. Perhaps it is public speaking that bothers you, or maybe it's arguing with your spouse or children. Whatever it is, recognizing what makes you uneasy will help you to address it immediately. Soothing your mind every day will make addressing Illnesses feel more possible because you will be in a more balanced mindset regularly.

How can I balance my mind when I begin to feel uncomfortable or anxious?

You should know when you are emotionally imbalanced (this could be anything from feeling anxious at work to feeling overwhelmed in a relationship) and address the emotional state immediately. Perhaps it's going for a walk before a fight with your spouse is about to break out. Maybe it's meditation or prayer. If your uneasiness pertains to presentations at work, try concentrating on a positive statement (or an "I am" speech) before you are about to get in front of a large group. Whatever it is, know what it is that calms you and be sure to implement it as soon as you feel the "fight or flight" syndrome coming on.

Exercising the mind in a positive manner means not allowing yourself to be consumed by negativity. Just as you would not eat junk food before a long race, you should not feed your mind with rubbish when you're trying to maintain balance in a stressful situation.

We have already established that a balanced life begins with self-respect and self-love; however, its definition stems from your beliefs and your desires.

What makes you happy to get up in the morning? What makes you say, "Wow, this is going to be a good day!" What makes you say, "Today I will conquer my Illness!"

I will use myself as an example. To me, happiness means loving myself and loving the people in my life. It means enjoying my work, but having enough time to go to the gym several times a week and always getting a good night's rest. It means feeling good about myself every morning and pushing myself each day to obtain the goals that make the world a better place.

Ask yourself what your definition of happiness is. Assuming there is self-love and self-respect (because we must love ourselves before we can properly love others), ask yourself, "What is my definition of happiness?"

Understanding what makes you happy and working towards this goal will trigger positive thoughts. Again, the whole idea of a balanced mindset is about understanding the power you have over your own mind. You have the ability to welcome the thoughts you would like to focus on versus those you want to dismiss. Simply put, when you choose to think positive thoughts, the universe will give you more positive things to think about. When you choose to think about negative thoughts, the universe will give you more things to think negatively about.

We have all experienced a bad day – the feeling we have when it seems as though nothing is going well. At work, we are frustrated and at home everyone seems miserable. You get up in the morning and you look and feel awful. You're edgy and irritable and it shows.

Now try to recall a really good day, one where you experienced quite the opposite feelings. You get up with a jump in your step and know the day will be good. You are smiling and it feels like the whole world is smiling back. You look good and it seems as though everyone is taking notice. The day is still full of its regular interruptions, but things are not getting under your skin. You are able to brush off negativity quite easily, and you are able to welcome all of the goodness that life has to offer.

How we handle good and bad days is an example of the power of your mind. We do not *have* good days and bad days – we only interpret them as such. *We*, alone, call it a "bad" day. And the reason a bad day is interpreted as "bad" is because you are welcoming negative thoughts. Rather than isolating a particular incident we internalize the feeling and wrap our perceptions around it. All of a sudden what started as an argument with your spouse turns into, for example, road rage or a dispute at work, and you end up feeling frustrated with your kids before you put them to bed. The entire day is ruined because you welcomed a whirlwind of negative thoughts.

The same is true of positive thinking. If you consume yourself with positive thinking, you will draw more happiness back into your life, or even into the current day. The law of attraction applies to the universe as a whole, and it also applies to this scenario: if we are drawn towards happiness, happiness will come to us.

Exercising the body is the next component in the healing process. It is the idea that what you feed your body and how you choose to nourish and care for it will have an impact not only on the longevity of your life, but also on your quality of life.

As a nation, we are inundated with high-fat, sodium-filled foods. We eat foods that are pumped with chemicals and steroids while they lack vitamins and nutrients. This unhealthy habit is compounded by the twenty-first century mentality that everything we need is found on the computer or television; unfortunately, what this means is that we also fail to notice how little physical exercise we are getting.

As a result, millions of North Americans are overweight, over-stressed, sleep-deprived, and at risk of suffering deadly diseases because of their chosen lifestyle. We are more educated than ever before, and yet it is as though our intellect has hindered our health and well-being. We have the World Wide Web at our finger-tips; however, we also have fast food restaurants on every block. As we have gotten smarter, we have most definitely gotten fatter.

So how do we stop this deadly eating pattern? How do we choose foods that will help us recover from our Illnesses and feel good about ourselves?

The answer is simple: Know about what you eat and understand the effects of these foods.

If you truly want to be happy and understand that your diet is largely connected to your well-being, you will educate yourself as to what it is you are putting in your body. Take the necessary steps to learn what your body needs and how to keep it energized and properly fueled. Understand approximately how many calories are in the foods you eat, and be keenly aware of what your caloric intake should be for each day. Ensure that your day's activities offset the food (and the types of food you put into your body for the day).

Some quick rules to remember:

- Read all labels before you purchase food at the grocery store.
- Do not ever go to the grocery store hungry.
- Carry healthy snacks with you at all times – raw almonds, fruits, vegetables or wraps are all good options (stay away from high sugar meal replacement bars).
- Eat small portions approximately every three hours (six meals per day). Do not skip meals!
- Do not eat in front of the television.
- Be conscious of what you are eating while you are eating it and chew each bite 10 times on each side of your mouth before you swallow.
- Minimize your intake of canned or packaged goods.
- Store low-fat desserts in the freezer – if you really want it you will have to be willing to wait for it to thaw.
- Keep a journal of everything you eat.
- Stay away from alcoholic beverages as best you can – a sugary alcoholic drink can have as many calories as a meal!
- Try eating your meals on smaller plates for portion control.
- Do not completely eliminate food groups – ever! Our bodies need the right proportion of non-starchy carbohydrates, good fats, and healthy, low-fat proteins.
- If you are concerned with your body composition, toss your scale and measure your success by how you feel and how your clothes fit.

Aside from nourishing yourself with the right foods, keeping yourself active throughout your life, especially while coping with an Illness, is paramount to your overall well-being. Though it may be the last thing we want to do on a bad day (and in some cases even on a good day), it is the best thing for you. I'm of the opinion that exercise should be the first form of treatment if at all possible.

When you undergo an Illness, start by moving yourself. Get up and put yourself into gear!

Exercising the body through resistance training and cardiovascular activity releases endorphins that create a balanced mindset and helps with relaxation and mental health. In essence, maintaining an active lifestyle can actually trigger happiness and positive thinking. Working out can help cure your Illness. You will feel more relaxed, self-confident, and you may even like what you see in the mirror!

Some benefits of maintaining a healthy, active lifestyle include:

- Mood elevation
- Stress reduction
- Elevated self-esteem and self-confidence
- Better sleeping habits
- Healthy weight loss
- Increased feelings of sexual arousal
- Lowered risk of heart disease, high blood pressure, obesity, type-2 diabetes, and many other life-threatening diseases.

The last component of Project Elinor is focused on working toward your spiritual health. To some, this means growing closer to your particular faith, while others see this as an opportunity to draw from their own Inner Wisdom. Regardless of your degree of religious practice, this last section focuses on your spirituality and inner strength.

No matter how you define your spirituality, it is important to take time each day to reflect on something larger than yourself. This can be done through prayer, meditation, or simple reflection.

Soon after my mother passed I recall an afternoon when my father and I went to lunch. Like an innocent child would ask his mother, my father asked me "if Mom was okay." Essentially, he was asking me if there was a heaven because he wanted to know where she was. For the first time in my life, my dad did not have all the answers, and like a little boy asking a parent, my dad turned to me. It was then that I realized more clearly than ever before, how important it is that we have a connection to our own spirituality.

Similar to my father, when we first experience an Illness, we want to question everything. Particularly when coping with an Illness caused by the death of a loved one, where answers cannot readily be found, we might wrestle with questions constantly. Our ability to search within ourselves for answers that have no obvious responses can aid in the recovery process.

At first it may be a bit uncomfortable to sit and reflect, but with time it will get easier and you will learn to trust your Inner Self. You need to learn to trust this process. Sit up straight in a quiet room. Wear comfortable clothes. Begin by thinking about a blank white screen. Allow no other thoughts into your mind and be calm and still. Allow yourself to breathe deeply.

Once you feel your thoughts have settled, ask yourself a question – like my father did – and consciously clear your mind while waiting for an answer. If you find your mind wandering, remind yourself that this time is strictly for you. It's not time to analyze and critique things. This time is devoted to your personal reflection. Be conscious of what thoughts enter your mind as your Inner Self tries to answer your question. What is God, or your Intuition, telling you?

The more comfortable we are with this ritual, the more assured we are by the answers that come through during reflection. There is a reason certain things just "feel right." When we are truly connected with ourselves, the truth and answers that we are searching for always lie within reach. It is a wonderful world of confidence that we enter when we trust our Inner Selves. The ever-changing world is not so frightening when we are balanced from within.

Gratitude is central to healthy spirituality. Building on the notion that we are one small piece of the larger picture of life, we must learn to be thankful and appreciative for being given our part in the universe. Being thankful means being happy about who we are and what we have, despite our Illnesses.

Take a couple minutes before you go to bed each night to state what you are grateful for. Even at our lowest moments, there are things in our lives that we can be thankful for. Maybe it's your heath or your family – whatever it is, tell yourself, or your God, about your appreciation.

What you will find in doing this exercise daily is that when your spirit is smiling, it feels like the whole world is smiling back. By maintaining your gratitude to the world and wholeheartedly feeling as though there is always something to be happy about (and there *is* always something to be happy about!), you inevitably begin to balance your Inner Self.

Too often we go about our daily lives rushing around taking little notice of the beautiful things around us. We fall victim to depression or anger because of our Illnesses, and we seldom stop to appreciate the good things life has to offer. I like to remind my clients that life is complicated, but that embracing these complexities allows us to have fully rounded souls. Take the time to look around you: What do you see outside of your Illness? What do you see inside of yourself? The more in touch you are with your spiritual side, the more connected you are to your own soul – the core of your very being.

Whatever method you choose to develop your emotional well-being, it is important to connect with yourself daily. Search within yourself constantly. Learn to trust yourself and your instincts. Understand that we are all just little pieces of a massive world and be sure you do not lose sight of that. You are not the only one suffering, and you are not the only one recovering. You are not any more or less important than the person living next to you, and your Illness is no more or less paralyzing. Take your Illness and embrace it because it makes up the "you" that you are supposed to be. There is a reason you are going through this, but relinquish the desire to seek that answer. Let it be and focus on healing.

Our Illnesses will weave in and out of our lives forever. Some of us are affected several times. Our suffering makes us human – it helps us discover who we are and what we can become. We all suffer from Illnesses; however, it's what we make out of them and how we choose to grow from them that is important.

When do you know you have overcome your Illness?

You are healed when you truly feel at peace with your life and everyone in it. The recovery happens when you allow your mind to be more powerful than your Illness. When you view your loss as an integral piece of the person you are, and a necessary stepping stone toward the happier and healthier life you have *chosen* to live. It is then that you have overcome your Illness.

MY JOURNAL

www.ingramcontent.com/pod-product-compliance
Lightning Source LLC
Chambersburg PA
CBHW051422280526
45785CB00003B/1122